Researching Health Promotion

Edited by Jonathan Watson
and Stephen Platt

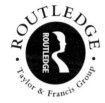

London and New York

First published 2000
by Routledge
11 New Fetter Lane, London EC4P 4EE

Simultaneously published in the USA and Canada
by Routledge
29 West 35th Street, New York, NY 10001

Routledge is an imprint of the Taylor & Francis Group

Typeset in Times by Taylor & Francis Books Ltd
Printed and bound in Great Britain by St Edmundsbury Press, St
Edmundsbury, Suffolk

British Library Cataloguing in Publication Data
A catalogue record for this book is available from the
British Library

Library of Congress Cataloging in Publication Data
Researching health promotion / edited by Jonathan Watson and
Stephen Platt.
p. cm.
Includes bibliographical references and index.
1. Health promotion–Research. I. Watson, Jonathan, 1960–II. Platt,
Stephen.
RA427.8 .R47 2000
613'.072–dc21   99–046625

ISBN 0 415–21590–0 (hbk)
ISBN 0 415–21591–9 (pbk)

Contents

List of illustrations   ix
Notes on contributors   xi
Acknowledgements   xv

1 **Connecting policy and practice: the challenge for health
   promotion research**   1
   JONATHAN WATSON AND STEPHEN PLATT

**PART I
Fresh thinking**   21

2 **Repositioning health promotion: research implications**   23
   ERIO ZIGLIO

3 **Think globally, act locally: what are the implications
   for health promotion and research?**   38
   HILARY WHENT

4 **A critical approach to lifestyle and health**   54
   THOMAS ABEL, WILLIAM C. COCKERHAM
   AND STEFFEN NIEMANN

PART II
Methodological challenges   79

5 Postmodernism and health promotion:
   implications for the debate on effectiveness   83
   DALE WEBB AND DAVID WRIGHT

6 Evidence and the evaluation of a community-level intervention:
   researching the Gay Men's Task Force initiative   102
   PAUL FLOWERS, JAMIE FRANKIS AND GRAHAM HART

7 Implementation of health promotion policy in Norwegian
   municipalities   125
   ELISABETH FOSSE

8 Does health economics do health promotion justice?   142
   JANINE HALE

PART III
Good practice   157

9 The creation of gendered spaces as a medium for
   sexual health promotion among young people in Peru   161
   MARCELO RAMELLA AND JENNIFER ATTRIDE-STIRLING

10 A theoretically based, cross-cultural study of infant
   feeding in new mothers and their partners   183
   VIVIEN SWANSON AND KEVIN POWER

11 Peer-led HIV prevention among gay men in London
   (the 4 gym project): intervention and evaluation   207
   JONATHAN ELFORD, LORRAINE SHERR,
   GRAHAM BOLDING, MARK MAGUIRE AND FRASER SERLE

12 Falling on deaf ears? Responses to health education messages
    from the Birmingham Untreated Heavy Drinkers Cohort   231

    CICELY KERR, JENNY MASLIN, JIM ORFORD, SUE DALTON,
    MARIA FERRINS-BROWN AND ELIZABETH HARTNEY

13 Older people's perceptions about health behaviours over
    time in Ireland: implications for health promotion   254

    ANNE MACFARLANE AND CECILY KELLEHER

    Index   270

Illustrations

Figures

1.1	UK policy connections	10
2.1	A credible approach	26
2.2	Type of investment	26
3.1	Features of a sustainable environment	40
3.2	Sustainable development and health	42
3.3	Sustainability indicators	46
4.1	Weber on lifestyle	59
4.2	Lifestyle, life chances, life conduct	63
4.3	Health lifestyle	64
4.4	Donkey analogy	65
4.5	Correspondence analysis: deprivation and health orientations	71
4.6	Correspondence analysis: deprivation and health behaviour	73
10.1a	Agreement with the breast-feeding views of partner, own mother, friends, midwives and people in general for Scottish breastfeeders, Scottish bottlefeeders, and Greek breastfeeders and combined feeders	194
10.1b	Importance of the views of partner, own mother, friends, midwives and people in general, for Scottish breastfeeders, Scottish bottlefeeders, and Greek breastfeeders and combined feeders	195
11.1	Criteria for a well-designed evaluation according to the Cochrane Collaboration (1993)	209
11.2	Invervention	214
11.3	The 4 gym project logo	215

12.1	Main barrier model	244
12.2	Attention sub-system	245
12.3	Damage sub-system	247
12.4	Individual differences sub-system	248
12.5	Barrier sub-system	248

Tables

4.1	List of indicators	69
6.1	Overview of research structure (1995–1999)	105
6.2	Demographic and recruitment characteristics	110
7.1	Research focus in a decision perspective and a process perspective on implementation	129
7.2	Ideologies and strategies at the central level	133
7.3	Differences between community projects and environment health projects	137
10.1	Percentage of women breast-feeding post-natally (on leaving hospital) for selected countries	184
10.2	Characteristics of mothers and their partners in the Scottish and Greek samples	191
10.3	Positive and negative breast-feeding and bottle-feeding beliefs for breast-feeding and bottle-feeding mothers and their partners in Scotland, and breast-feeding and combined-feeding mothers and their partners in Greece	193
11.1	Baseline survey: number of questionnaires distributed and returned	218
11.2	Timetable for the intervention and its evaluation	219
11.3	Evaluation: primary outcomes to be compared at each survey point	222
11.4	Baseline survey: social and demographic characteristics of the study population	226
11.5	Baseline survey: men reporting unprotected anal intercourse in previous three months	227
12.1	Characteristics of the health education focus sub-sample	236
13.1	Demographic and socio-economic profile of interview study participants	257
13.2	Reported determinants of health: sub-categories and their sub-classifications	259

Contributors

Professor Thomas Abel, Unit for Health Research, Institute for Social and Preventive Medicine, University of Bern, Switzerland

Dr Jennifer Attride-Stirling Researcher, Social Psychology Department, London School of Economics

Graham Bolding, Research Assistant, Department of Primary Care and Population Sciences and Royal Free Centre for HIV Medicine, University College London

Professor William C. Cockerham, Professor of Sociology, Medicine and Public Health, Department of Sociology, University of Alabama

Sue Dalton, Research Associate and current Project Manager of the Birmingham Untreated Heavy Drinkers Project, Drinking Research Group, School of Psychology, University of Birmingham

Dr Jonathan Elford, Senior Lecturer in Epidemiology, Department of Primary Care and Population Sciences and Royal Free Centre for HIV Medicine, University College London

Maria Ferrins-Brown, Research Interviewer, Birmingham Untreated Heavy Drinkers Project, Drinking Research Group, School of Psychology, University of Birmingham

Dr Paul Flowers, Research Associate, MRC Social and Public Health Sciences Unit, Glasgow

Elisabeth Fosse, Research Fellow, Research Centre for Health Promotion, University of Bergen, Bergen, Sweden

Jamie Frankis, MRC Social and Public Health Sciences Unit, Glasgow

Janine Hale, Research Fellow, Health Economist, Health Promotion Wales

Professor Graham Hart, Associate Director, MRC Social and Public Health Sciences Unit, Glasgow

Elizabeth Hartney, former Research Associate for the Birmingham Untreated Heavy Drinkers Project, Drinking Research Group, School of Psychology, University of Birmingham

Professor Cecily Kelleher, Professor of Health Promotion, Centre for Health Promotion Studies, National University of Ireland

Cicely Kerr, formerly Research Interviewer with the Birmingham Untreated Heavy Drinkers Project, now West Midland Local Research Co-ordinator for the UK Alcohol Treatment Trial, Drinking Research Group, School of Psychology, University of Birmingham

Dr Anne MacFarlane, Researcher, Centre for Health Promotion Studies, National University of Ireland

Mark Maguire, HIV Prevention Office, Health Promotion Service, St Pancras Hospital, London

Jenny Maslin, previously Research Interviewer with the Birmingham Untreated Heavy Drinkers Project, now as research psychologist working with the Combined Psychosis and Substance Use (COMPASS) programme in Birmingham

Steffen Niemann, Assistant, Unit for Health Research, Institute for Social and Preventive Medicine, University of Berne.

Professor Jim Orford, Professor of Clinical and Community Psychology, School of Psychology, University of Birmingham

Professor Stephen Platt, Director, Research Unit in Health and Behavioural Change, Medical School, University of Edinburgh

Professor Kevin Power, Professor of Clinical Psychology, Anxiety and Stress Research Centre, Department of Psychology, University of Stirling

Marcelo Ramella, SaRA Project Manager, Social Psychology Department, London School of Economics

Fraser Serle, HIV Prevention Office, Health Promotion Service, St Pancras Hospital, London

Dr Lorraine Sherr, Senior Lecturer in Health Psychology, Department of Primary Care and Population Sciences and Royal Free Centre for HIV Medicine, University College London

Dr Vivien Swanson, Lecturer, Anxiety and Stress Research Centre, Department of Psychology, University of Stirling

Professor Jonathan Watson, Director of Research and Evaluation, Health Education Board for Scotland, Edinburgh

Dale Webb, Research Fellor, Wessex Institute for Health Research and Development, University of Southampton

Hilary Whent, Senior Researcher, Health Education Authority, London

Dr David Wright, Primary Care Research Co-ordinator, Primary Medical Care, University of Southampton

Dr Erio Ziglio, Health Promotion and Investment Programme, World Health Organization, Regional Office for Europe, Copenhagen, Denmark

Acknowledgements

We are very grateful to Heather Gibson and Fiona Bailey at Routledge for their support and help during the production of this book. We are also grateful to staff at the Research Unit in Health and Behavioural Change and the Research & Evaluation Division at the Health Education Board for Scotland, for their helpful suggestions and comments. Thanks are also due to Jenie Glover at RUHBC for ensuring that the text was properly formatted and for chasing down missing references etc. from the various contributors.

Chapter 1

Connecting policy and practice

The challenge for health promotion research

Jonathan Watson and Stephen Platt

Introduction

We are witnessing a number of significant political, economic and social transformations that are bringing about important changes in the conception and organisation of health and social care. The World Health Organization has for some years seen itself as addressing the 'new social, political, economic and environmental challenges' of the close of the century (WHO 1991). One consequence of these transformations has been the privileging of public health and the improvement or promotion of health. However, in this chapter, we argue that there has been little coherent attempt to align theoretical developments in health promotion research to shifting policy agendas.

Building on the Lalonde Report (Lalonde 1974), the Alma Ata Declaration on Primary Health Care (1978), and the Health For All 2000 Strategy (1981), the First International Health Promotion Conference in Ottawa in 1986 (WHO 1986) focused on the potential for widening the role of health promotion to encompass work with communities and organisations as well as with individuals. To accomplish this it identified five strategies for health promotion action: building healthy public policy, creating supportive environments, strengthening community action, developing personal skills and reorientating health services. More recently, the Fourth International Conference in Jakarta endorsed this approach and identified a number of key action points to carry the health promotion agenda forward into the twenty-first century:

- promoting social responsibility for health (i.e. private and public sectors should pursue policies and practices that avoid harm to health)

- increasing investments for health development (i.e. using a truly multi-sectoral approach and prioritising the needs of particular groups)
- consolidating and expanding partnerships for health (i.e. between the different sectors and at all levels of society)
- increasing community capacity and empowering the individual in matters of health (i.e. health promotion by and with people, not on or to people)
- securing an infrastructure for health promotion (in particular, through targeting settings such as schools and workplaces).

(WHO 1997)

The agenda established in Ottawa, and developed subsequently through conferences in Adelaide (healthy public policy), Sundsvall (supportive environments) and Jakarta (partnership), is mirrored in the UK by fresh Government initiatives on the future of the National Health Service (DoH 1997, SODoH 1997), new health policy (DoH 1999, SODoH 1999) and action on social inclusion (Social Exclusion Unit 1998, The Scottish Office 1999). Overall, the nineties have witnessed a radical shift in the policy agenda from a neo-liberal ideology, which targets the privatisation of health by devolving responsibility for managing risk to the individual (Petersen 1997: 194), to the new public health agenda, which seeks to address the socio-economic determinants of health in addition to the existing lifestyle focus.

The evolving nature of health promotion has implications for health promotion research and related research agendas. By health promotion research, we mean research that services the needs of health promotion by, for example, helping to refine the practices and approaches of health promotion. Relevant questions include: what works, in what circumstances and with whom? (Health Education Board for Scotland 1999, Wimbush in press). By contrast, research on (or of) health promotion, may be concerned with developing critiques of health promotion practice or studying the values base of policy and practice (Nettleton and Bunton 1995: 41–3, Thorogood 1992). These should not be discrete enterprises. Specifically, we need to be able to assess scientific knowledge relevant to health promotion across a variety of research paradigms/ disciplines; and decide when existing basic research in a particular area supports a transition to more applied research (health promotion research). Both encompass a wide range of disciplines, among them epidemiology, anthropology, psychology, organisational and political science and sociology, that do not always sit comfortably side by side.

This volume draws on papers presented at, and reflections prompted by, the First UK Health Promotion Research Conference, held in Edinburgh in April 1998. The conference was organised against the backdrop of this evolving international agenda and recent UK Government policy initiatives. As such, it provided a timely opportunity to explore the main challenges for health promotion research in the twenty-first century.

Two key themes recurred throughout the conference: the nature of knowledge and the meaning of evidence in health promotion. Epistemological debate on these themes is unavoidable, in part because the health promotion field is shaped by, and interacts with, complex phenomena and processes, and in part because there is a diversity of expertise informing research, policy and practice.

The nature of knowledge

The terrain for basic and applied health promotion research is broad, ranging from population-level prevention activity, through individual-level interventions to action on the structural and cultural determinants of health. While recognising the multi-faceted nature of health, its production and maintenance, the tendency has been to assume that health promotion practice should encompass a similarly broad sweep. Whitelaw *et al.* (1997) have argued that this tendency is unhelpful because it masks tensions between competing paradigms and agendas. Specifically, they warn that 'the creation of ... "global" health promotion models could inhibit constructive debate around alternative perspectives on health' (480). They conclude by noting that 'permanent tensions' exist that need not necessarily be resolved. They identify three initial areas for attention: professional and political matters, technical and methodological dilemmas, and research questions. The challenge for practitioners is how they manage these tensions in order to deliver action that addresses contemporaneous policy agendas (ibid.: 487–8). This chapter raises issues for consideration in respect of the focus and nature of research within which specific research questions require framing.

The shift in the policy agenda can be attributed to a range of influences that can be encapsulated under three headings: governance in late modernity, health inequalities and agency. These provide a set of 'lenses' through which the development of theoretical domains in health promotion research and practice might profitably be focused and developed. The notion of 'theoretical domains' was developed by Dean (1993) with respect to the problem of linking theory and methods in population health research. According to Dean, 'theoretical domains may be thought of as developmental frameworks for elaborating causal processes to build bodies of knowledge in substantive areas' (ibid.: 29). In this context, problem solving is concerned with the complexity of dynamic relationships among components of a domain rather than the 'prediction of global truths' or probable outcomes. Dean's concept has an intuitive resonance for an emergent health promotion field, because it not only situates theory in real world contexts but it gives a role to methods in the building of theory (ibid.: 30–32). Elsewhere, Noack (1997) and Platt (1997) have identified that in many health intervention studies the underlying theoretical models are non-existent or poorly defined. Rather by default, health promotion continues to rely largely on models and theories of health behaviour originally published in the 1970s (Wallston *et al.* 1978, Bandura 1977, Ajzen and Fishbein 1977, Becker 1974, Bem 1972, Rogers and Shoemaker 1971). Overall, there has been little coherent attempt to align theoretical development to shifting policy agendas (notable exceptions include Gillies 1998, Gillies and McVey 1996, Whitelaw and Williams 1994; Ziglio – see Chapter 2). Similarly, the manifest good intentions of health promotion have acted as a barrier to the development of an informed critique (for exceptions see especially Seedhouse 1996 and Bunton *et al.* 1995).

Governance in late modernity

Giddens argues that we are living through a period of 'late modernism' characterised by rapid social change which profoundly 'affects pre-existing social practices and behaviour' (Giddens 1991: 16; see also Giddens 1990). This is set against a context of broad social transformations of globalisation, the advent of new cyber and information technologies, the changing nature of the disease burden, ageing populations and the rise of consumer culture (Burrows *et al.* 1995, Featherstone and Burrows 1995, Featherstone 1991). These circumstances are said to give rise to chronic uncertainty and heightened notions of risk. In these circumstances, scientific knowledge is constructed around risk and the expertise required to manage risk (Petersen 1997, Beck 1992, Giddens 1991). However, as Lupton notes: 'The risks which are selected by a society as requiring attention may ... have no relation to "real" danger but are culturally identified as important' (Lupton 1995: 80). Critically, as Lupton later asserts, 'the notion of internally imposed risk has yet to be fully critiqued for its political and moral dimension' (ibid.: 81) and it is this perception of risk, derived from clinical medicine and epidemiology, which tend to inform health promotion.

Arguably, such developments in the policy agenda can be seen as opening up new opportunities for surveillance (Armstrong 1995, 1983). This perspective is informed by Foucault's work (1979, 1973) which gave an impetus to the identification and examination of new forms of governance and concomitant techniques of surveillance (Watson in press, Petersen 1997, Lupton 1995, Armstrong 1995, Bunton 1992; see also Armstrong 1983 on epidemiology and general practice). However, the particular technique of surveillance of interest in this context is that of health economics. For, ironically, the boost given to health promotion by Ottawa and recognition of the key role of health promotion in Government health policy statements in the early nineties (DoH 1992, SOHHD 1992) coincided with global concerns about containing the escalating costs of health care (Macdonald 1996, Anderson 1984). Through a recognition that many health problems were related to individual lifestyles (Anderson 1984), the issue of cost containment became conflated with a concern to manage the consequences of risk. In this milieu, a key element of the new health care culture was that decisions about how to improve health and health care should be informed by evidence of need and especially evidence of effectiveness and cost-effectiveness. That is, given finite resources, choices have to be made between competing uses of health care resources. For example, a recent policy review summarised the cost-effectiveness of treatment and prevention of coronary heart disease. The authors concluded that 'although not all forms of prevention are successful or represent value for money, there is evidence that well-designed and targeted programmes, particularly those concerned with smoking and diet, can have a significant effect on reducing risk factors, and represent good value for money in terms of life gained' (SODoH 1996: 65).

Although such assessments appear to make a *prima facie* case for health economics, there is debate regarding its value to health promotion (Craig and Walker 1996, Tolley *et al.* 1996, Burrows *et al.* 1995, Cohen 1994). Burrows *et al.* (1995: 241) state that the organisation and delivery of health care is increasingly realised through the concept of 'value for money'. Most interestingly, they develop an argument that the hegemony of health economics within health systems is explained by an organisational need for 'ontological security' that 'the rhetoric of rationality' provides in an era (late modern) of incessant change and disruption. Nevertheless, they conclude that health economics is unable to adequately cope with the task of evaluating health promotion. This is significant, in part, because it challenges us to pose the question 'on whose terms is something effective' and what are valid endpoints in health. Crucially, there is a need to consider the consequences of pursuing community health promotion. In particular, what are valid endpoints or outcomes of such activity? Certainly, the measurement of community-level change poses major methodological problems but, as Sheill and Hawe (1996) have argued, the key issue is the extent to which one believes that community-level change is adequately captured by adding up measures of cognitive or behavioural change across individuals. Valid endpoints for community health development programmes might include, for example, non-health or indirect health outcomes, such as sense of community, community empowerment, and community competencies that impact upon the social, cultural, economic, environmental and political determinants of health. It is imperative that the methods we use fully capture the desired effects of a programme. Failure to do so may result in misleading practitioners/policymakers as to their value.

Health inequalities

A second influence on the development of a new policy agenda for health promotion has been the rediscovery of the determinants or 'root causes' of excess morbidity and premature mortality which are external to individuals and provide the context for their behaviour and actions. Several widely used models of health (Dahlgren and Whitehead 1991, Labonte 1998, Evans and Stoddart 1994) illustrate the range of contextual factors, including the economic, psychosocial, cultural and physical environments, that shape overall population health and inequalities in health relating to socioeconomic status, gender, age and other social positions.

In the UK, the Independent Inquiry into Inequalities in Health (Acheson Report 1998) was guided by a socio-economic model of health. This model emphasised the impact of over-arching general, societal, living and working conditions, which themselves influence the quantity and quality of social and community networks, which in turn condition health lifestyle attitudes and behaviours. The Report notes the evidence of long-standing and widening gradients in mortality between the higher and lower socio-economic groups in the UK and prioritises the implementation of policies which will reduce income inequalities and lead to the redistribution of resources to those who find themselves, unavoidably, outside the labour market. The authors of the Report are adamant that the policy emphasis must move 'upstream', from the de-contextualised individual to the social and economic structure: 'We consider that without a shift of resources to the less well off, both in and out of work, little will be accomplished in terms of a reduction of health inequalities by interventions addressing particular "downstream" influences' (Acheson Report 1998: 33).

This view is reinforced by the growing evidence of a strong relationship between income inequality and premature mortality within developed societies (see, especially, Wilkinson 1996). One plausible explanation for this relationship is the relative strength or weakness of the psychosocial fabric, in particular, features of everyday life which engender and promote social cohesion. 'Social capital', which has been defined by Putnam (1995: 67) as 'the features of social organisation such as networks, norms and social trust that facilitate co-ordination and collaboration for mutual benefit', is the concept now widely employed to capture this societal attribute. It is hypothesised that more egalitarian societies generate higher levels of social capital which in turn reduce health inequalities and increase life expectancy. Gillies (1998) argues that the notion of social capital revitalises *social* approaches to public health and health promotion, since it permits examination of the processes whereby social connections operating through different networks can act as a buffer against the negative health impact of relative (as well as absolute) deprivation.

Agency

A final cluster of factors may be seen to operate around assertions of agency under late modern conditions. These have included the influence of the main social and self-help movements in the twentieth century (women, civil rights, independent living) and the emergence of community development and the Internet pioneers (Rootman *et al.* 1998, Bunton and Macdonald 1992, Green and Kreuter 1991, Green and Raeburn 1990). Giddens (1984: 9) has described agency as follows:

> Agency refers not to the intentions people have in doing things but to their capability of doing those things in the first place ... Agency concerns events of which an individual is the perpetrator, in the sense that the individual could, at any phase in a given sequence of conduct, have acted differently.

Popay *et al.* (1998: 637) argue that current theory and research on health inequalities (and by implication, policy and practice) are limited because they do not readily address the relationship between structure and agency and, in particular, the possibility for, and determinants of, creative human agency. Between individuals and their capacity to act, they identify a number of 'mediating concepts'. These include autonomy, control and identity and 'the central role of narratives in the "construction" of self-identity'. In particular, they cite the work of Somers (1994), who argues that the experience of social action is constituted through narratives. They end by suggesting that, in the context of health inequalities, there is a 'strong case for looking at people's perceptions of "episodes" in their lives and the ways in which these may orientate or fail to orientate action at the individual or collective level'.

The tension between structure and agency

These overlapping influences which have propelled health promotion and public health back to centre-stage also illustrate the key tension that lies at the heart of health promotion and which has yet to be resolved by its advocates, namely the relationship between determinism and self-will (Kelly and Charlton 1995) or, in social science terminology, structure and agency (Giddens 1984, 1979). Contemporaneously with Giddens, McQueen argued that the relationship between an individual and society was perhaps the most important in social sciences research. He asks:

is there actually some kind of interaction which takes place between [the individual and society] … if one takes seriously the current view that it is the context in which health behaviours occur, which must be studied, then the interplay between the societal and the individual is the most critical problem in contemporary research.

(McQueen 1986: 293)

Giddens has been the foremost advocate of structuration theory which highlights the structuring of social relations across time and space in the context of everyday life, the lifecourse of an individual and institutions. In this context, health promotion, like anthropology, occupies a 'cultural borderland' (Gantly 1994) where different perspectives, sectors, groups, research paradigms, practice and policy agendas come together and/or conflict. For some this is a weakness of the health promotion project (Kelly and Charlton 1995) while for others it is a strength (Burrows *et al.* 1995). This confusion is not resolved by the meta-conceptualisation of health promotion as 'involving a diverse set of actions focused on the individual or environment which through increasing control ultimately leads to improved health or well being' (Rootman *et al.* 1998: 7).

What is clear is the need to distinguish between health promotion as a process and the improvement of health as an outcome. In this sense, the distinctive contribution of health promotion may be its ability or otherwise to facilitate linkages between structure and agency. Figure 1.1 highlights the principles underpinning UK Government policy thinking in the late 1990s which, in turn, may provide a map for a policy–practice connected evidence base. A recent expert panel concluded that health promotion specialists were the only players in a position to 'make the links between [and within] health improvement programmes, Local Agenda 21, healthy living centres, regeneration partnerships, health action zones' (Rogers *et al.* 1997).

The meaning of evidence

Internationally, the Cochrane Collaboration and, in the UK, the Centre for Reviews and Dissemination at York and the Epi-Centre in London, have developed and implemented a particular approach to sifting and presenting systematic reviews of effectiveness. This approach has involved the adoption of a hierarchy of evidence,

Figure 1.1   UK policy connections

1   Equity of access – improving access to public services
2   Raising standards – improving the quality of public services
3   Integration and coordination – of policies and services
4   Partnership working
5   Community participation – active citizenship
6   Decentralisation – decision-making devolved to local level
7   Understanding – of best practice and what works
8   Openness/transparency – of Government and public services
9   Prevention of problems – through early or upstream action
10   Sustainability – mainstreamed rather than one-off initiatives

which emphasises the randomised controlled trial as a gold standard for evaluation design, followed by other non-randomised studies such as quasi-experimental designs, cohort and case control designed interventions and descriptive studies using surveys and practitioner reports. The emergence and application of qualitative methods to evaluation was largely ignored, although currently being addressed. This will not immediately resolve the question of what should constitute appropriate and reliable evidence in health promotion. The experience of trying to use reviews published to date is that they provide an insufficient basis upon which to make an appraisal of options to inform the development of practice or policy. Reviewers often conflate the effectiveness of an intervention with the effectiveness or 'quality' of its evaluation (Research and Evaluation Division 1996). Within the hierarchical system described above, the effectiveness of an activity is directly linked with the form of its evaluation and evidence from studies conforming to these criteria is prioritised. By contrast, there is a need to develop a system for dealing with findings from the multi-level, multi-method studies that are increasingly being advocated by those concerned to demonstrate the impact of health promotion at individual, organisational and community levels.

An example is provided by Brännström *et al.* (1994) who sought to develop a framework to assess the outcomes of community-based intervention programmes for the promotion of cardiovascular health at local level. Their outcome assessment took account of individual and community change and included assessment of community participation (using questionnaires, focus groups, public meetings and in-depth interviews); a socio-epidemiological study (focusing on medical/behavioural outcomes); a key informants study (comprising in-depth interviews); content analysis of the mass media; and description of social, cultural and political change (using participant observation, key informants and written documents). Although this represented a relatively complex research strategy for measuring outcomes, it allowed the researchers to analyse different aspects in the intervention process and in so doing to attempt to contextualise the behavioural outcomes in the cumulative and dynamic interplay of structure and agency to which Chapman (1993) refers. This broader approach to evidence is one that draws on available theory, research findings and professional and lay knowledge, recognising that different sources of evidence inform policy and are required to translate policy into practice and to assess the impact of such action (Nutbeam 1998, Speller *et al.* 1997, Tones 1997, Ham *et al.* 1995, Chapman 1993, Hirschon-Weiss and Wittrock 1991).

Evaluating health promotion

The effectiveness and cost-effectiveness of health promotion interventions are under increasing scrutiny in the new evidence-based cultural climate within the health sector in the UK and elsewhere. While there is some concern about the extent to which expectations relating to the success of health promotion practice are more pronounced than those relating to clinical practice, the problem most commonly identified by researchers is the unwillingness of funding and commissioning agencies to accept the validity and viability of non-experimental evaluation strategies. We would argue that methodological pluralism should embrace a range of evaluation designs as well as multiple and mixed methods. Again, it is important not to misunderstand the point being made here. There is (probably growing) recognition that randomised controlled trials and quasi-experiments have an important place in the armoury of the health promotion evaluation researcher, provided that the importance of rigorous process (as well as outcome) assessment is seen as integral to the research design. In this context, Ann Oakley makes a forceful and challenging contribution to the debate about the value of experimentation and social interventions. In two recent articles (1998a, 1998b) she has argued that experts who block the use of randomised controlled trials, in determining what works in social interventions, ignore a considerable history of experimentation within social science. Taking the specific case of health promotion, Oakley suggests that this stance is, in part, a product of practitioners' search for a distinct professional identity (1998b: 84). Her bottom line, equally critical of medical as well as health promotion practitioners, is that

> What randomised controlled trials offer in the social domain is exactly what they promise to medicine: protection of the public from potentially damaging uncontrolled experimentation and a more rational knowledge about the benefits to be derived from professional interventions.
>
> (Oakley 1998a: 1,242)

Nutbeam has challenged the position adopted by Oakley on three counts (Nutbeam 1999). First, that in all the cases cited by Oakley, the unit of intervention was the family or individuals. By contrast, many contemporary social interventions are seeking to alter the risk profile in populations. Second, the interventions were relatively simple to measure and control in contrast to complex multi-layered interventions common in existing health promotion programmes. Third, that maintaining a separation between 'control' and 'intervention' populations over long time periods is difficult (Nutbeam 1999: 944). Nutbeam's position is reflected in current WHO guidance on evaluation (Rootman et al. 1997). From such a perspective it could be argued that the major challenge to all stakeholders in health promotion research (but particularly researchers and funders/commissioners) is to make the fullest use of existing non-experimental designs and devise new strategies which capture evolution and change in process and address the problem of causal attribution (i.e. how outcomes can be linked to the intervention) in real-life, real-time situations.

From a practitioner perspective, a related consideration in the design and methods for health promotion research is that care should be taken to ensure that there is an adequate fit with health promotion principles and practice. In particular, there is a case for saying that the use of non-participatory approaches that serve to disempower and alienate individuals or communities should be avoided, while those that exemplify partnership and inclusion should be pursued. Related notions of community involvement, openness and transparency underpin many of the recent policy statements emanating from the UK Government. In a sense, participatory research should not be seen as a separate method or one alternative among many, rather it is about ensuring that the research questions posed are relevant, the methods understandable and the findings meaningful (Institute of Health Promotion Research/B.C. Consortium for Health Promotion Research 1995).

Notwithstanding this and despite the seeming incompatibility of the cases advanced by Oakley and Nutbeam, they do appear to overlap. Arguably, they agree that randomised controlled trials are appropriate in evaluating the effectiveness of relatively 'straight-line' interventions, e.g. the use of nicotine replacement therapy in primary care settings. Similarly, they appear to agree on the need properly to take account of qualitative data in establishing the effectiveness of multi-level interventions. One might also presume that they would recognise legitimate concerns about the tendency to focus on the quality of outcome evaluations and an attendant lack of concern for the quality of the actual intervention. Elsewhere, Fraser and Whitelaw (1998) make a case for the importance of an 'integrated, iterative evaluation programme which gives a convincing account of the intervention, enabling outsiders to understand and appreciate why things were done as they were and what came of it'. They go on to note that 'it is unrealistic to expect one methodology to address all the legitimate questions one might ask of a programme in order to assess its worth'. They use the example of the SHARE evaluation (an MRC-funded teacher-delivered sex education programme for 13 to 15-year-olds) as an illustration of the use of integrated methodologies (including the randomised controlled trial).

That said, there is broad agreement among practitioners, researchers and policy-makers that the endpoint of health promotion action is, or rather should be, the improvement of health and well-being, rather than the reduction of morbidity and mortality or the limitation of health damaging 'lifestyle' behaviours, such as smoking or alcohol misuse. Despite extensive discussion in recent years about the need to develop appropriate indicators to measure positive health outcomes, progress has been disappointingly slow. In addition to the technical issues that have to be resolved (e.g. testing of new indicators and establishment of their psychometric properties), there is evidence to suggest that some funders/commissioners and policy-makers remain to be convinced about this reorientation. It is important to give reassurance that traditional epidemiological and health education outcomes are not being ignored or downplayed. Rather, the latter are conceptualised as intermediate outcomes within a socio-ecological model of health which emphasises the social, cultural, economic and physical environment, together with genetic endowment, as fundamental determinants of population health.

In the introduction to a recent anthology of health promotion, Helena Restrepo commented that 'the accumulation of knowledge is a process of small incremental growth' (Pan American Health Organisation 1996). In one sense, the plethora of reports, articles and guidelines on or about health promotion contradict this view. Yet, the PAHO anthology represented an acknowledgement of the importance of improving the quantity and quality of research dissemination and implementation. The successful implementation of research into practice is a measure of progress in realising the rhetoric of evidence-based practice. Kitson *et al.* (1998: 149) suggest that successful implementation is a function of three core elements: level and nature of evidence; context or environment in which research is placed; and method or way in which the process is facilitated. Contrary to much current dissemination practice, they do not privilege the first of these elements. Rather, the three elements are given equal recognition. However, they acknowledge that their conceptual framework does not account for how innovative practice (i.e. with limited or no research evidence) is successfully adopted.

In the spirit of the recent UK White Papers on public health (SODoH 1999, DoH 1999), the development of more productive partnerships between researchers, policy-makers and practitioners should be given high priority. Researchers are urged to be more proactive in their efforts, targeting key opinion leaders in policy and practice, as well as in their own academic community. A successful research dissemination strategy will incorporate an analysis of the needs of diverse constituencies and stakeholders, and ensure that feedback on research findings is produced in appropriate and accessible formats. One major problem, which requires immediate and urgent attention, is lack of indicators that capture this broader impact of research upon policy and practice. The current, almost exclusive, emphasis upon outputs in published books and academic journals when considering achievement in the university research sector (the Research Assessment Exercise in the UK) is manifestly inadequate in this regard. Another issue to be addressed is the provision of adequate training for researchers so that they can acquire the skills and competencies demanded by a wider dissemination role.

Conclusion

An optimistic view is that the antagonisms between different epistemological and methodological paradigms within health (promotion) research are beginning to dissolve with growing recognition that more pluralistic and synthesising approaches are both feasible and desirable. Certainly, what concerns funders and commissioners is the clarity of the aims and objectives of a specific research proposal and the specification of a methodological strategy likely to deliver stated outcomes. Above all, they seek rigour and quality. The task of the research community is to ensure the highest possible standards, drawing on the full range of qualitative and quantitative methods, as appropriate.

Finally and perhaps inevitably, in any field there is a lead and lag relationship between theory (or understanding how something works) and action. In health promotion, theory has lagged behind action. In consequence, it has become increasingly difficult to account for how and in what ways action is linked to (or takes forward) policy. This is evident in the relationship between the issues addressed in Part I (Fresh thinking) and Part II (Methodological challenges) of this volume, when compared to the issues that are the focus in Part III (Good practice). By the time of the next UK Health Promotion Research Conference in 2000, those of us working in this field need to have taken steps to reduce the gap between theory and practice, to encourage a broader disciplinary engagement with health promotion around key theoretical domains and ensure a better fit between research, practice and policy.

References

Acheson Report (1998) *Independent Inquiry into Inequalities in Health*. London: The Stationery Office.

Ajzen I., Fishbein M. (1977) 'Attitude-behaviour relations: a theoretical analysis and review of empirical literature'. *Psychological Bulletin* 84: 888–918.

Anderson R. (1984) 'Health promotion: an overview'. In: L. Baric (ed.) *European Monographs in Health Education Research*. Edinburgh: Scottish Health Education Group.

Armstrong D. (1995) 'The rise of surveillance medicine'. *Sociology of Health and Illness* 17: 393–404.

—— (1983) *Political Anatomy of the Body: Medical Knowledge in Britain in the Twentieth Century.* Cambridge: Cambridge University Press.

Bandura A. (1977) *Social Learning Theory*. London: Prentice Hall.

Beck U. (1992) *Risk Society: Toward a New Modernity*. London: Sage.

Becker M. (ed.) (1974) 'The health belief model and personal health behaviour'. *Health Education Monographs* 2: 1–146.

Bem D. (1972) 'Self-perception theory: an alternative interpretation of cognitive dissonance phenomena'. In: L. Berkowitz (ed.) *Advances in Experimental Social Psychology* 6. New York: Academic Press, pp. 1–62.

Brännström I., Persson L., Wall, S. (1994) 'Towards a framework for outcome assessment of health intervention'. *European Journal of Public Health* 4: 125–30.

Bunton R. (1992) 'More than a woolly jumper: health promotion as social regulation'. *Critical Public Health* 3: 4–11.

Bunton R., Macdonald G. (1992) *Health Promotion: Disciplines and Diversity*. London: Routledge.

Bunton R., Nettleton S., Burrows R. (1995) 'Sociological critiques of health promotion'. In: R. Bunton, S. Nettleton, R. Burrows (eds) *The Sociology of Health Promotion: Critical Analyses of Consumption, Lifestyle and Risk*. London: Routledge.

Burrows R., Bunton R., Muncer S., Gillen K. (1995) 'The efficacy of health promotion, health economics and later modernism'. *Health Education Research* 10: 241–9.

Chapman S. (1993) 'Unravelling gossamer with boxing gloves: problems in explaining the decline in smoking'. *BMJ* 307: 429–32.

Cohen D. (1994) 'Health promotion and cost-effectiveness'. *Health Education Research* 9: 281–7.

Craig N., Walker D. (1996) 'Choice and accountability in health promotion: the role of health economics'. *Health Education Research* 11: 355–60.

Dahlgren G., Whitehead M. (1991) *Policies and Strategies to Promote Equity in Health*. Stockholm: Institute for Future Studies.

Dean K. (1993) 'Integrating theory and methods'. In K. Dean (ed.) *Population Health Research: Linking Theory and Methods*. London: Sage, pp. 9–36.

Department of Health (DoH) (1992) *Health of the Nation*, London: HMSO, Cm 1968

—— (1997) *The New NHS: Modern, Dependable*. London: The Stationery Office, Cm 3807

—— (1999) *Saving Lives: Our Healthier Nation*. London: The Stationery Office, Cm 4386

Evans R., Stoddart G. (1994) 'Producing health, consuming health care'. In: R. Evans, M. Barer, T. Marmor (eds) *Why Are Some People Healthy and Others Not: The Determinants of Health of Populations*. New York: Aldine De Gruyter, pp. 27–64.

Featherstone M. (1991) 'The body in consumer culture'. In: M. Featherstone, M. Hepworth., B. Turner (eds) *The Body: Social Processes and Cultural Theory*. London: Sage, pp. 170–96.

Featherstone M., Burrows R. (1995) 'Cultures of technological embodiment: an introduction'. *Body and Society* 1: 1–20.

Foucault M. (1979) *Discipline and Punish: The Birth of the Prison*. Harmondsworth: Penguin.

—— (1973) *The Birth of the Clinic*. London: Tavistock.

Fraser E., Whitelaw A. (1998) 'From polemic to narrative: deconstructing the RCT'. Paper presented at *Working Together for Better Health* International Conference, Cardiff, 23–25 September.

Gantly M. (1994) 'The qualitative and the quantitative: an anthropological perspective on research methods'. *Critical Public Health* 5: 27–32.

Giddens A. (1979) *Central Problems in Social Theory: Action, Structure and Contradiction in Social Analysis*. London: Macmillan.

—— (1984) *The Constitution of Society: Outline of the Theory of Structuration*. Cambridge: Polity Press.

—— (1990) *The Consequences of Modernity*. Cambridge: Polity Press.

—— (1991) *Modernity and Self-Identity: Self and Society in the Late Modern Age*. Cambridge: Polity Press.

Gillies P. (1998) 'Social capital and its contribution to public health'. In: E. Ziglio, D. Harrison (eds) *Social Determinants of Health: Implications for the Health Professions*. Genoa: Italian National Academy of Medicine, pp. 46–50.

Gillies P., McVey D. (1996) *HEA Research Strategy 1996–1999*. London: Health Education Authority.

Green L., Kreuter M. (1991) *Health Promotion Planning: An Educational and Environmental Approach*. Mountain View, CA: Mayfield.

Green L., Raeburn J. (1990) 'Contemporary developments in health promotion: definitions and challenges'. In: N. Bracht (ed.) *Health Promotion at the Community Level*. London and Newbury Park, CA: Sage.

Ham C., Hunter D., Robinson R. (1995) 'Evidence-based policy making'. *BMJ* 310: 71–3.

Health Education Board for Scotland (1999) *Research for a Healthier Scotland: The Research Strategy of the Health Education Board for Scotland*. Edinburgh: HEBS.

Hirschon-Weiss C., Wittrock B. (1991) 'Social sciences and modern states'. In: P. Wagner, C. Hirschon-Weiss, B. Wittrock., H. Wollmann (eds) *Social Sciences and Modern States: National Experiences and Theoretical Crossroads*. Cambridge: Cambridge University Press.

Institute of Health Promotion Research/B.C. Consortium for Health Promotion Research (1995) *Study of Participatory Research in Health Promotion: Review and Recommendations for the Development of Participatory Research in Health Promotion in Canada*. Vancouver, BC: The Royal Society of Canada.

Kelly M., Charlton B. (1995) 'The modern and the postmodern in health promotion'. In: R. Bunton, S. Nettleton, R. Burrows (eds) *The Sociology of Health Promotion: Critical Analyses of Consumption, Lifestyle and Risk*. London: Routledge, pp. 78–90.

Kitson A., Harvey G., McCormack B. (1998) 'Enabling the implementation of evidence-based practice: a conceptual framework'. *Quality in Health Care* 7: 149–58.

Labonte R. (1998) *A Community Development Approach to Health Promotion*. Edinburgh: Health Education Board for Scotland/Research Unit in Health and Behavioural Change, University of Edinburgh.

Lalonde M. (1974). *A New Perspective on the Health of Canadians*. Ottawa: Health and Welfare Canada.

Lupton D. (1995) *The Imperative of Health: Public Health and the Regulated Body*. London: Sage.

Macdonald G. (1996) 'Where next for evaluation?' *Health Promotion International* 11: 171–3.

McQueen D. (1986) 'Health education research: the problem of linkages'. *Health Education Research* 1: 289–94.

Nettleton S., Bunton R. (1995) 'Sociological critiques of health promotion'. In: R Bunton, S. Nettleton., R. Burrows (eds) *The Sociology of Health Promotion: Critical Analyses of Consumption, Lifestyle and Risk*. London: Routledge, pp. 41–58.

Noack H. (1997) 'Review and evaluation of health promotion'. Working paper prepared for *New Players for a New Era: Leading Health Promotion into the Twenty-First Century*. Fourth International Conference on Health Promotion, Jakarta, Indonesia, 21–25 July.

Nutbeam D. (1999) 'Oakley's case for using randomised controlled trials is misleading' (letter). *BMJ* 318: 994.

—— (1998) 'Evaluating health promotion: progress, problems and solutions'. *Health Promotion International* 13: 27–44.

Oakley A. (1998a) 'Experimentation and social interventions: a forgotten but important history'. *BMJ* 317: 1,239–42.

Oakley A. (1998b) 'Experimentation in social science: the case of health promotion'. *Social Sciences in Health* 4: 73–88.

Pan American Health Organisation (1996) *Health Promotion: An Anthology*. Washington, DC: WHO.

Petersen A. (1997) 'Risk, governance and the new public health'. In: A. Petersen, R. Bunton (eds) *Foucault, Health and Medicine*. London: Routledge, pp. 189–206.

Platt S. (1997) 'Evaluation in health education/promotion: a guide to best practice'. Paper presented at First Annual HEBS/RUHBC Research Meeting, 5 November.

Popay J., Williams G., Thomas C., Gatrell T. (1998) 'Theorising inequalities in health: the place of lay knowledge'. *Sociology of Health and Illness* 20: 619–44.

Putnam R. (1995) 'Bowling alone: America's declining social capital'. *Journal of Democracy* 6: 65–78.

Research and Evaluation Division, Health Education Board for Scotland (1996) 'How effective are effectiveness reviews?' *Health Education Journal* 55: 359–62.

Rogers A., Popay J., Williams G., Latham M. (1997) *Health Variations and Health Promotion: Insight from the Qualitative Literature*. London: Health Education Authority.

Rogers E., Shoemaker F. (1971) *Communication of Innovations: A Cross Cultural Approach* (2nd edn). New York: The Free Press.

Rootman I., Goodstadt M., Potvin L., Spingett J. (1998) *Towards a Framework for Health Promotion Evaluation*. Copenhagen: World Health Organization Regional Office for Europe.

Scottish Office, The (1999) *Social Inclusion: Opening the Door to a Better Scotland*. Edinburgh: The Scottish Office.

Scottish Office Department of Health (SODoH) (1996) *Coronary Heart Disease in Scotland: Report of a Policy Review*. Edinburgh: Scottish Office Department of Health, Public Policy Unit.

—— (1997) *Designed to Care: Renewing the National Health Service in Scotland*. Edinburgh: The Stationery Office.

—— (1999) *Towards a Healthier Scotland*. Edinburgh: The Stationery Office.

Scottish Office Home and Health Department (SOHHD) (1992) *Scotland's Health: a Challenge to Us All*. Edinburgh: HMSO.

Seedhouse D. (1996) *Health Promotion: Philosophy, Prejudice and Practice*. Chichester: John Wiley

Sheill A., Hawe P. (1996) 'Health promotion, community development and the tyranny of individualism'. *Health Economics* 5: 241–7.

Social Exclusion Unit (1998) *Bringing Britain together: A National Strategy for Neighbourhood Renewal*. London: The Stationery Office.

Somers M. (1994) 'The narrative constitution of identity: a relational and network approach'. *Theory and Society* 23: 605–49.

Speller V., Learmonth A., Harrison D. (1997) 'The search for evidence of effective health promotion'. *BMJ* 315: 361–3.

Thorogood N. (1992) 'What is the relevance of sociology for health promotion?' In: R. Bunton, G. Macdonald (eds). *Health Promotion: Disciplines and Diversity*. London: Routledge, pp. 42–65.

Tolley K., Buck D., Godfrey C. (1996) 'Health promotion and health economics'. *Health Education Research* 11: 261–64.

Tones K. (1997) 'Beyond the randomised outcome trial: a case for judicial review'. *Health Education Research*, 12: i–iv.

Wallston K., Wallston B., Devellis R. (1978) 'Development of the multidimensional health locus of control (MHLC) scales'. *Health Education Monographs* 6: 160–170.

Watson J. (in press) *Male Bodies: Culture, Health and Identity*. Milton Keynes: Open University Press.

Whitelaw A., McKeown K., Williams J. (1997) 'Global health promotion models: enlightenment or entrapment?' *Health Education Research* 12: 479–90.

Whitelaw A., Williams J. (1994) 'Relating health education research to health policy'. *Health Education Research* 9: 519–26.

World Health Organization (WHO) (1986) *Ottawa Charter*. Geneva: WHO.

—— (1997) *The Jakarta Declaration: On Leading Health Promotion into the 21st Century*. Geneva: WHO.

World Health Organization (WHO) Regional Office for Europe (1991) *Introducing the Lifestyle and Health Department*. Copenhagen: WHO

Wilkinson R. (1996) *Unhealthy Societies: The Affliction of Inequality*. London: Routledge.

Wimbush E. (in press) 'Developing a monitoring and evaluation framework for health promotion'. *Evaluation*.

Part I

Fresh thinking

In Chapter 2, Erio Ziglio considers the research implications of the World Health Organization's revised policy for health, Health 21, with its emphasis upon 'upstream' socio-economic determinants and an 'Investment for Health' approach which places health improvement and the reduction of health inequalities at the centre of public policy development. In particular, he calls for the expanded use of modelling to identify the specific public policies which affect health; an improved effort to understand the obstacles to intersectoral collaboration within policy agencies; more sophisticated research on the bridges and barriers to successful investments for health; further developments in audits of health promotion resources in order to assess infrastructural capacity for investing in health; research on the bureaucratic environment and the complexities of decision-making; development of long-term measures of public investment impact; undertaking inventories of health promotion assets and resources; and devising new measures to capture collective, synergistic effects of a healthy community on economic and social development. This constitutes a formidable and challenging agenda for the research community, which the author himself recognises.

Relatedly, Hilary Whent (Chapter 3) assesses the implications of sustainability for health promotion. Agenda 21, the international development plan produced at the Rio Earth Summit in 1992, takes forward the concept of sustainable development, which brings together a whole range of interrelated issues: protection of the environment, improvement of quality of life and economic development. Community participation in policy decisions and action is a key principle that underpins the plan. Health promotion policy and sustainable development intersect in many areas. At a local level a significant Local Agenda 21 (LA21) movement is emerging among local authorities, with the majority claiming commitment to the process. While some are repackaging current activities as LA21, many are creating new arrangements and initiatives and genuinely engaging local people. It is argued that stronger links should be made between health promotion and LA21 strategies. There is a concern that LA21 work tends to be narrowly focused on environmental issues without capturing the true concept of sustainability. For health promotion, LA21 offers the opportunity to take a much broader based approach to promoting health and working towards community participation.

In Chapter 4 Thomas Abel, William Cockerham and Steffen Niemann argue that the lifestyle approach can be criticised for its reductionist perspective, leading to an overemphasis on behavioural aspects and on the individual. Indeed, many earlier lifestyle studies in health research have neglected or downplayed the interplay of behaviour, on the one hand, and structural and cultural context, on the other. The traditional risk factor paradigm has inadequately reduced the meaning of the term lifestyle to a single relevant behaviour (or, at best, set of such behaviours). This misuse of the term lifestyle, along with an insufficiently developed theoretical foundation, has resulted in an increasingly vague and diffuse understanding of the lifestyle approach. Through analysis of current lifestyle discourse, Abel and colleagues identify three types of lifestyle concepts: general lifestyles and their impact on health, health relevant lifestyles, and health oriented lifestyles. Having clarified basic issues, they present a new concept that combines structural and behavioural aspects in the formation of health relevant lifestyles based on a Weberian understanding of lifestyles as the product of the complex interplay between life chances and life conduct. Lifestyle is thus reconceptualised in a way that goes beyond the current debate of structural determinism *versus* free choice.

Chapter 2

Repositioning health promotion
Research implications

Erio Ziglio

Introduction

The World Health Organization's original strategy for health promotion was developed in the mid-1980s and articulated in the Ottawa Charter of 1986 (WHO 1984, 1986). After more than a decade it is time to take stock and ask how the latest developments and scientific findings can help take the whole issue of health promotion forward into the twenty-first century. The major stimulus for this review comes from the accumulated evidence that conditions have changed dramatically in Europe since the mid-1980s. It has become imperative to assess the new circumstances and ask what kind of health promotion strategy is needed to deal most effectively with the emerging issues.

Europe itself has changed. Within a few short years, the European region of WHO has expanded its recognised 'membership' from thirty to over fifty countries. This has brought about massive social as well as political changes, and at such a rapid rate that the societies have had no time to adjust (Makara 1994, Unicef 1977, Ziglio 1993, 1998b). In some cases, these changes have been accompanied by increasing outbreaks of armed conflict, including instances of the most bitter civil wars to be experienced in Europe for many decades.

The global economic changes have been especially challenging in Europe, where the additional transitional forces among newly independent states have created high levels of uncertainty and anxiety about the future. Problems related to economic development (or lack of it) have been common in many countries, and in today's Europe there is a rising proportion of the population living in poverty and experiencing unemployment or job insecurity, in the West as well as the East.

While chronic unemployment has plagued several areas of Europe since the oil crises of the 1970s, the unemployment trends in the 1990s have affected a wider sweep of people who have never before experienced joblessness (Cornia and Paniccia 1995). These include skilled workers, technicians, sales people, managers, administrators and civil servants. Furthermore, unemployment rates as high as 15 to 20 per cent in some European countries do not give the full picture (Cornia 1997). Increasing trends towards under-employment and job insecurity have added to the worsening situation.

The nature of the challenges to public health have changed and new phenomena are appearing. For example, the demographic and mortality crises in the East of the European region are unprecedented, other than in times of famine or war. Between 1989 and 1994, both birth and marriage rates fell by up to 40 per cent in several Eastern European countries (Cornia 1997). Over the same period, male death rates in Russia dramatically increased from such causes as cardiovascular disease and violence, while life expectancy declined to below retirement age (WHO 1998d). Widening inequalities in health within countries remain a trend of worrying concern throughout Europe.

Health promotion, thinking and action have to progress and develop to take on board these wide-ranging changes (Levin and Ziglio 1997). Based on the concept and principles embodied in the Ottawa Charter, a strategy for health promotion is needed which matches the new circumstances and rises to these challenges.

Refocusing upstream

An effective modern strategy of health promotion rests on two lines of analysis: first, a reassessment of the major health challenges facing Europe together with their root causes, and second, an examination of the current policy environment to assess how best it might be influenced.

From the reassessment, it is becoming clear that the root causes of Europe's health problems lie in the massive changes that have taken place in the social and economic conditions in recent decades. In policy terms, there is a need to refocus 'upstream' to the wider determinants of health in the social and economic policy environment and how these might be addressed (Ziglio et al. 1998).

An assessment of how policy in sectors beyond health care might be influenced suggests that more emphasis should be put on the idea of health being an investment (Hancock 1982, Kickbusch 1997). The economic and social development of European countries will depend to a significant extent upon effective measures to promote and sustain the health of the peoples of the continent (WHO 1996a). A healthier population is both more contented and more productive; an unhealthy population, on the other hand, is an indication of wasted human potential and unnecessary suffering which could add to the atmosphere of discontent and unrest in a society.

The Investment for Health approach

Health is a crucial social and personal resource that needs nurturing – that needs investment. But it is also true that if we invest in ways that secure positive health and well-being, we also bring about social and economic benefits for the whole country/community. (Ziglio 1998a). By contrast not all social and economic investment promotes health (WHO 1998b). The key is to identify those investments which do. In doing this, it is imperative that health promotion is implemented through an Investment for Health approach that tackles the roots of the main causes of ill-health in a credible, effective and ethical manner (Ziglio 1998a). This means developing strategies which are based on, and tackle, key determinants of health. Such determinants are mainly linked to social and economic factors influencing life conditions. Lifestyles should be seen as patterns of behaviour heavily influenced by life conditions.

Figure 2.1 helps visualise a credible approach to health promotion. It provides a pragmatic framework for health promotion implementation by means of an Investment for Health approach, whereas Figure 2.2 gives an idea of the type of investment (public/individual) pertinent to different components of health promotion programmes and policies.

Figures 2.1 and 2.2 show that a robust implementation of a health promotion strategy needs to be based on a good balance of programmes and policies (see Figure 2.1) and to make use of a portfolio of Investment for Health (see Figure 2.2). Health promotion has to be pursued, and increasingly perceived, as an innovative modern strategy which, in addition to health benefits to the population, contributes to 'healthy' social and economic returns for a nation, in a sustainable and equitable way. This message is embodied

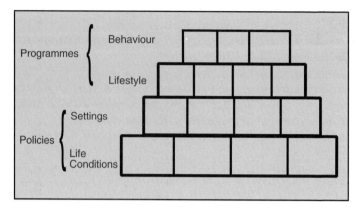

Figure 2.1   A credible approach

Type of Investment	Life Conditions	"Settings"	Lifestyles	Behaviour
Which Type of Investment? **Where do we make our Investment?**				
Development Measures Public/Private	✓✓✓✓	✓✓✓	✓✓	✓
Individual Measures	✓	✓	✓✓	✓✓✓

Figure 2.2   Type of investment

in the Jakarta Declaration and has found its place in the renewed Health For All policy of the WHO Regional Office for Europe, known as 'Health 21' (WHO 1997c, 1998b).

Kickbusch (1997) argues that there are at least three key questions which need to be addressed in developing a strong and credible health promotion strategy:

- where is health promoted and maintained in a given population?
- which investment and strategies produce the largest population health gains?
- which investment and strategies help reduce health inequities and are in line with human rights?

These questions are at the heart of the Investment for Health approach (Ziglio 1998b). Such an approach attempts to address an additional question. Namely, which investment provides added value to social and economic development in an equitable and sustainable manner resulting also in high health returns for the overall population? (Ziglio 1998a). Only a very few of the reforms underway in many European countries are currently attempting to place these questions on the table (Ziglio 1998b, Saltman and Figueras 1997). It is in the practical attempt to address the above health promotion related questions that the Investment for Health approach has begun to take shape.

Investment for Health is an approach for optimising the health promoting impact of development, namely, the result of public policies and private sector initiatives including, for example, education, labour, income maintenance, health care, housing, agriculture, tourism and transport. The Investment for Health approach involves identifying relevant policy attributes; considering factors that may enhance or inhibit policy change; assessing change options that offer benefits both to health goals and the primary intent of that specific policy sector; and planning the political process of achieving the necessary legislative, regulatory, financial, organisational or educational changes (Ziglio 1998a). Thus, Investment for Health is not a new concept. It is a pragmatic approach to implement the concept and principles of health promotion in practice.

Seen in this light, health promotion is an investment in the future social and economic development of a country. The 'Investment for Health' approach is the way in which the European Office of the World Health Organization is pushing the health promotion agenda forward. The ideas underpinning this approach can be summarised in five key principles:

- improving and maintaining health is an investment
- health investments must be made on the basis of the determinants of population health

- investment in health implies reorientation of health services and overall social and economic development
- investments should be compared for population health impact, both in terms of need reduction and health assets maximisation
- health investments must reduce inequities and be compatible with human rights.

The WHO/Euro programme

What is needed at an international level to reorientate thinking and initiatives in health promotion towards these new principles? The WHO Investment for Health programme aims to create a European advocacy infrastructure and tested policy tools for positioning health promotion as an investment strategy linked to social and economic development in European member states. In order to ensure this, the programme has prioritised four key areas:

1   the formation of a *European Committee for Health Promotion Development*, the purpose of which is to provide within the region a top level committee which is able to give authoritative advice on national policies, structures and effective practices of Investment for Health;
2   the provision of new investment *appraisal services* to enable European countries to identify their health assets and at the same time support healthy, sustainable and equitable economic and social development;
3   the setting up of a number of carefully selected Investment for Health *demonstration projects* aiming at testing different options in the use of policy measures (e.g. educational, managerial, fiscal, regulatory, etc.), to secure and sustain an investment strategy for the promotion of health;
4   the preparation of a policy-relevant set of publications and an overall investment for health *communication strategy*. The aim here is to foster innovation, provide materials, ideas and practical experiences at the cutting edge of policy development for the promotion of health.

Research implications

It has been pointed out above that Investment for Health is essentially a pragmatic approach to the implementation of sustainable and credible policies for the promotion of health. Several lessons have already been learned and new research issues are coming to the forefront. The approach is a relatively new field of policy action. It draws upon a wide range of theories and disciplines. It is believed that the research implications outlined below need and will attract much attention in the years to come.

Research on major social/economic determinants of health

This has not been historically an area of traditional epidemiologic and demographic research used as a basis for planning public health interventions. Even though it is conventional wisdom that exigencies of social/economic environment powerfully affect all aspects of development, the ethos and practice of public health have implicitly viewed health as linked primarily to epidemiologic, behavioural or clinical factors, independent of economic and other social trends and conditions (Levin *et al.* 1994, Evans *et al.* 1994). Indeed, the commitment to reduce health risk factors (e.g. behaviour) rather than attention to risk conditions (e.g. environment, poverty) has severely limited the effectiveness of efforts to promote population health (Bartley *et al.* 1997, Blane *et al.* 1996, Chu 1994, WHO 1995a, Mustard 1996, Marmot 1998).

The modelling of economic and social trends can help clarify which aspects of public policy sectors are mainly associated with specific threats to the public health. It is important that an investment strategy to improve health takes special care to assess (with as much accuracy as data will allow) those public policies and other aspects of overall development which affect health. A miscalculation here could be costly both in wasted resources and reduced credibility to the investment process itself. Here is where innovations in modelling the relationship of economic/social factors to population health status can help pinpoint investment options (health promoting interventions) and estimate their relative benefits. We are at a research 'frontier' with this application of model building, but the modelling strategy to predict trends and indicate investment options is a well-established market development tool.

Now we come to the crux of the matter, where there are many unanswered questions, both substantive and methodological. To strengthen public policy's favourable impact on population health will require negotiations around incentives that compensate for fiscal or other technical dislocations or provide equal value exchanges. Incentives also must take into account and mediate between some-times conflicting interests within a given policy sector or between sectors with overlapping remits (WHO 1996c, 1997a). Hierarchical decision-making structures within policy agencies (ministries, depart-ments) present additional barriers in so much as they may block 'horizontal' or trans-departmental communication and the collabo-ration necessary to implement the policy change (WHO 1995b). Selecting investment options is one thing; selling them is another. Our experience is deficient in those processes although, again, there is a parallel literature as investment strategies operate in market endeavours. We need our own data here; our own experience-rated strategies that can only derive from on-the-ground demonstrations or specific appraisals of investment opportunities of the kind WHO have been undertaking in Italy, Spain, Hungary, Slovenia and Germany (WHO 1995b, 1996a, 1996c, 1997b). This experience must be now analysed and prepared for publication and dissemination that can encourage further trials.

Research on policy change

Are there principles or 'rules' that predict the policy change process? Or put another way, can we predict or describe the factors which contribute to and/or block successful investments? There is clearly a need to generalise from our experience with the investment strategy although it is unlikely that we shall achieve 'one size fits all' principles.

Policy science is not an exact science (Wildavski 1979, Brewer and de Leon 1983, Milio 1981). Furthermore, myriad cultural and temporal variables create unique circumstances that defy full repli-cation of the process from state to state. Nevertheless, some impressions may emerge as strategic as well as ethical guidelines especially as they relate to ensuring equity, transparency and sustainability. The entire Investment for Health process needs objec-tive third party oversight to achieve a useful level of generalisability. After all, at this point we are operating with a patchwork of policy development and social change theories as well as 'borrowed' tech-nologies from policy science and organisational development (Senge 1990, Vedung 1997, Weiss 1998). To encourage health promotion specialists to adopt the Investment for Health approach, it is essen-tial that they have an understanding of the whole as well as its component parts.

Research on infrastructure

What agency should take on the role of 'lead agency' for the Investment for Health approach, given that 'everybody's business quickly becomes nobody's business'? It is not altogether clear that the health ministry should always become the focal point (WHO, 1999). There are special considerations that will influence what agency emerges as the facilitator of the process. The first consideration is clearly having the competence and vision to formulate and implement a plan for intersectoral action. The second qualification is real and perceived political and disciplinary neutrality and the credibility and authority to intercede in policy development. Few ministries can claim such governmental high ground. The research questions then become how is an enabling mechanism designed (process being crucial) and implemented (accepted)?

These are perhaps questions for the political scientist to ask, but the answers will require an organised audit of resources such as the audit of health promotion resources undertaken in Slovenia by WHO (WHO 1996a). In that case, an independent focal point linked to all ministries but reporting directly to the parliament was recommended. The audit as a promising research tool in determining administrative structure for the investment process needs further practical testing and refinement (Ziglio and Hagard 1998).

Research on decision-making levels

An interesting question, which should receive a high research priority, is how do (or should) Investment for Health strategies vary according to governmental level: local, sub-regional, regional, national and global (Labonte 1998, WHO 1998c, 1999). Policy sector differentiation appears to increase with each successive step up in government jurisdiction. At the local community level intersectoral collaboration in sharing resources for 'common causes' seems to occur with little or no formal negotiations (WHO 1997a). This 'natural' investment process is worthy of study. What is the anatomy of trust among key players at that level? Does 'barter and exchange' play a role and how is accountability for multi-sectoral policy impact shared? Are there collateral benefits that result, such as enhancing local action networks (building social capital)? Clearly, the Investment for Health process will be shaped in part by the bureaucratic environment, particularly the complexities of decision-making (Ziglio

1998a). There are multiple levels of approval and fragmentation of internal consultation among domains of expertise and 'need to know' interest groups. At each level of governance, one can expect a different constellation of stakeholders with varying power and authority. It can be expected, as well, that negotiation networks and style of negotiating will require adaptations in the investment process. Research on these questions is of interest to several disciplines: policy science, sociology, organisational behavior, anthropology, social psychology and interpersonal communication (Ziglio 1991, Levin and Ziglio 1996, 1997).

Research on impact

As a general concept, Investment for Health enjoys *prima facia* acceptance as logical and self-evident. There is overwhelming evidence that multiple public policies, as well as private sector initiatives, conspire for good or for bad to powerfully affect population health. Evaluation of the investment concept is, therefore, not so much a matter of providing evidence of cost benefits (except in noticeable exceptions such as the value of 'sin taxes') but in matters of cost-effectiveness (Ziglio 1996). What investment methods are most effective and economical with regard to the expenditure of human resources, finance and time? Self-appraisal techniques are, of course, useful and can be strengthened by building into the investment process an internal audit that accounts for performance 'costs' at each stage of investment: e.g. criteria setting, selecting policies, isolating key aspects of policy, negotiating change (including choosing incentives), implementation (promulgating laws, regulations) and public acceptability (approval, compliance).

But to gain a wider level of acceptability among ministers, parliamentarians and public health practitioners we shall need to go beyond self-study and seek long-term measures of policy investment impact. There is precedent for example, for investment monitoring in the world of finance with established indicators of market performance. Public health has its indicators as well, but they are rarely linked to changes in public policies. This is an exciting area of development for evaluating health investment interventions (Ziglio 1996). We shall have to explore what the possibilities are for both direct evidentiary links and proxy links where direct measures of the impact of public and private sector policy changes on health are not yet practical.

Research on health promoting assets

A sensible approach to all public health interventions is to know, as far as possible, the total situation in which the index problem exists. Situation reports vary widely with some being limited to basic demographic and epidemiologic facts. Other situation reviews are more inclusive of economic, social and cultural data. For purposes of Investment for Health, however, the situation review must go even further to include an inventory of health promoting assets, decision-making structures and 'players', as well as the overall political climate and public capacity for involvement. Promoting health is a social undertaking and thus there needs to be an inventory of resources (and processes) that go well beyond those resources that are associated with a 'problem'. We must seek out those resources that contribute to the creation of health without a specific reference to a disease.

With such a broad perspective, it is easy to see the importance of setting criteria (or categories) for inclusion. Such an inventory can help reveal gaps in health promoting resources. It can identify policy and regulatory changes needed to fill those gaps or enhance equitable access to existing resources. Undertaking an assets inventory also can help in building networks to improve or sustain health promoting resources.

Establishing and maintaining a current assets inventory will require considerable research and development of observational instruments and protocols. Demonstrations have shown the value of even a modest, time limited effort. But at the same time these demonstrations highlight the need for more sophisticated approaches to inventoring health assets (WHO 1995b, 1996a, 1996c, 1997b).

Research on development

The impact (or contribution) of a healthy population to economic and social development is an idea which has received much less research attention than the reverse question of how social and economic factors and forces affect health (Draper et al. 1997, Omran 1979, Popay et al. 1980, WHO 1995a, 1997b, 1998b). This is understandable since we have incontrovertible evidence that, for example, there is a strong relationship between family income and disease prevalence (Whitehead 1994, Whitehead et al. 1998, Wilkinson 1996). The measurements of both the independent variable (income) and dependent variables (incidence/prevalence of specific diseases and injuries) are clear-cut and easily observed.

Health (not merely the absence of disease) is, on the other hand, more difficult to define as the independent variable since it includes such culturally sensitive notions as well-being, happiness, contentment, self-worth, creativity, growth and sense of security. There are proxy measures which are useful in defining health as the independent variable (Sen 1995). These include, for example, levels of capacity for work and play and effective human relations (increased social capital). But linking these individual attributes to individual and collective contributions to economic and social development is difficult except in limited ways (e.g. lower absence rate from work). What is needed are ways to account for these individual health attributes in a collective way in order to measure the total, synergistic effect of a healthy *community* on economic and social development. It is this measure of synergy that needs to go beyond summing the status of individuals. This is a major challenge to scientists in several disciplines who themselves must 'collectivise' their contributions to achieve an integrated strategy.

References

Bartley M., Blane D., Montgomery S. (1997) 'Health and the life course: why safety nets matter'. *BMJ* 314: 1,194–6.

Blane D., Brenner E., Wilkinson, R. (1996) *Health and Social Organization: Towards a Health Policy for the 21st Century*. London: Routledge.

Brewer G., de Leon P. (1983) *Foundations of Policy Analysis*. Homewood, IL: Dorsey.

Chu C. (1994) 'Integrating health and environment: the key to an ecological public health'. In C. Chu and R. Simpson (eds) *Ecological Public Health: From Vision to Practice*. Queensland, Australia: Watson Ferguson & Company.

Cornia G. (1997) *Labour Market Shocks, Psychosocial Stress and the Transition's Mortality Crisis. Research in Progress Number 4*. Helsinki: United Nations University, WIDER.

Cornia G., Paniccia R. (1995) *The Demographic Impact of Sudden Impoverishment: Eastern Europe during the 1989–94 Transition*. Florence: Unicef, International Child Development Centre.

Draper P., Best G., Dennis J. (1997) 'Health and wealth'. *Royal Society of Health Journal* 97: 121–6.

Evans R., Barcer M., Marmot T. (eds) (1994) *Why Are Some People Healthy and Others Not?* New York: Aldine De Gruyter.

Hancock T. (1982) 'Beyond health care: creating a healthy future'. *The Futurist* August: 4–13.

Kickbusch I. (1997) *Think Health: What Makes the Difference?* Address to the 4th International Conference on Health Promotion. Jakarta, Indonesia, 21–25 July 1997. Geneva: World Health Organization, HPR/HEP/4ICHP/BR/97.3.

Labonte R. (1998) 'Healthy public policy and the World Trade Organization'. *Health Promotion International* 13: 245–56.

Levin S., McMahon L., Ziglio E. (eds) (1994) *Economic Change, Social Welfare and Health in Europe.* Copenhagen: World Health Organization, Regional Office for Europe.

Levin S., Ziglio E. (1996) 'Health promotion as an investment strategy: considerations on theory and practice'. *Health Promotion International* 11: 33–40.

—— (1997) 'Health promotion as an investment strategy: a perspective for the 21st century'. In M. Sidell, L. Johns, J. Katz and A. Peberdy (eds) *Debates and Dilemmas in Promoting Health.* London: Macmillan.

Makara P. (1994) 'The effect of social changes on the population's way of life and health: a Hungarian case study'. In S. Levin, L. McMahon, E. Ziglio (eds) *Economic Change, Social Welfare and Health in Europe.* Copenhagen: World Health Organization, Regional Office for Europe, WHO Regional Publications, European Series No. 54.

Marmot M. (1998) 'Improving the social environment to improve health'. *Lancet* 351(1): 57–60.

Milio N. (1981) *Promoting Health Through Public Policy.* Philadelphia: F.A. Davis.

Mustard J. (1996) 'Health and social organization in health and social capital'. In D. Blane, E. Brunner, R. Wilkinson (eds) *Health and Social Organization.* London: Routledge.

Omran A. (1979) 'Changing patterns of health and disease during the process of national development'. In G. Albrecht, P. Higgins (eds) *Health, Illness and Medicine: A Reader in Medical Sociology.* Chicago: Rand McNally.

Popay J., Griffiths J., Draper P., Dennis J. (1980) 'The impact of industrialisation on world health'. In World Future Society (ed.) *Through the '80s: Thinking Globally Acting Locally.* Washington D.C.: World Future Society.

Saltman R., Figueras J. (1997) *European Health Care Reform. Analysis of Current Strategies.* Copenhagen: World Health Organization, Regional Office for Europe, WHO Regional Publications, European Series No. 79.

Sen A. (1995) *Mortality as an Indicator of Economic Success and Failure.* Florence: Unicef, Istituto degli Innocenti.

Senge P. (1990) *The Fifth Discipline – The Art and Practice of the Learning Organization.* New York: Doubleday.

Unicef (1997) *Children at Risk in Central and Eastern Europe: Peril and Promises.* Economies in Transition Studies, Regional Monitoring Report, No. 4. Florence: Unicef, International Child Development Centre.

Vedung E. (1997) *Public Policy and Programme Evaluation.* London: Transnational Publisher.

Weiss C. (1998) *Methods for Studying Programmes and Policies.* Upper Saddle River: Prentice Hall.

Whitehead, M. (1994) 'Counting the human costs: opportunities for and barriers to promoting health'. In Levin *et al.* 1994.

Whitehead, M., Dahlgren, G., Diderichsen, F. (1998) 'Social inequalities in health. What are the issues for health promotion?' Unpublished working document for the European Committee for Health Promotion Development. Copenhagen: World Health Organization, Regional Office for Europe, Health Promotion and Investment Programme.

Wildavski A. (1979) 'Speaking truth to power'. *The Art and Craft of Policy Analysis.* Boston: Little Brown.

Wilkinson R. (1996) *Unhealthy Societies.* London: Routledge.

World Health Organization (WHO) (1984) *Health Promotion: A Discussion Document on the Concept and Principles.* Copenhagen: World Health Organization, Regional Office for Europe.

—— (1986) *Ottawa Charter for Health Promotion.* Copenhagen: WHO, Regional Office for Europe.

—— (1995a) *Health in Social Development.* WHO Position Paper. World Summit for Social Development, Copenhagen, March 1995. Geneva: WHO.

—— (1995b) *Securing Investment for Health. Report of a Demonstration Project in the Provinces of Bolzano and Trento.* Copenhagen: World Health Organization, Regional Office for Europe, Health Promotion and Investment Programme.

—— (1996a) *Investment for Health in Slovenia.* Copenhagen: World Health Organization, Regional Office for Europe, Health Promotion and Investment Programme.

—— (1996b) *Investing in Health Research and Development.* Report of the Ad Hoc Comittee on Health Research Relating to Future Intervention Options. Geneva: World Health Organization.

—— (1996c) *Investment for Health in the Valencia Region: Mid-Term Report. Copenhagen: World Health Organization.* Regional Office for Europe, Health Promotion and Investment Programme.

—— (1997a) *Intersectoral Action for Health: Addressing Concerns in Sustainable Development.* Geneva: World Health Organization.

—— (1997b) *Investment for Health in Hungary.* Copenhagen: World Health Organization, Regional Office for Europe, Health Promotion and Investment Programme.

—— (1977c) *The Jakarta Declaration on Leading Health Promotion into the 21st Century*. Copenhagen: World Health Organization.

—— (1998a) *The World Health Report*. Geneva: World Health Organization.

—— (1998b) *Health 21 in the 21st Century*. European Health for All Series No. 5. Copenhagen: World Health Organization.

—— (1998c) *Public Health in Latvia – With Particular Reference to Health Promotion*. Copenhagen: World Health Organization, Regional Office for Europe, Health Promotion and Investment Programme.

—— (1998d) *Health in Europe*. Copenhagen: World Health Organization.

—— (1999) *Benchmark I: System Characteristics. The Verona Initiative – Investing for Health in the Context of Economic, Social and Human Development*. Copenhagen: World Health Organization, Regional Office for Europe, Health Promotion and Investment Programme.

Ziglio E. (1991) 'Indicators of health promotion policy: directions for research'. In B. Badura and I. Kickbusch (eds) *Health Promotion Research. Towards a New Social Epidemiology*. Copenhagen: World Health Organization, WHO Regional Publication No. 37, 55–83.

—— (1993) 'European macro trends affecting health promotion strategies'. WHO/EURO Working Paper. Copenhagen: World Health Organization, Regional Office for Europe, Health Promotion and Investment Programme.

—— (1996) 'How to move towards evidence-based health promotion interventions'. *Promotion and Education* 4(2): 29–33.

—— (1998a) 'Producing and sustaining health: the investment for health approach'. Key Note Speech, The Verona Initiative – Investing for Health in the Context of Economic, Social and Human Development. Copenhagen, Arena Meeting 1, Verona, Italy, October 14–17. Paper available through: World Health Organization, Health Promotion and Investment Programme.

—— (1998b) 'Key issues for the new millennium'. *Promoting Health The Journal of Health Promotion for Northern Ireland*. 2: 34–7.

Ziglio E., Hagard S. (1998) *Appraising Investment for Health Opportunities*. Copenhagen: World Health Organization, Health Promotion and Investment Programme.

Ziglio E., Levin L., Bertinato L. (1998) 'Social and economic determinants of health: implications for health promotion'. *Forum* (Special Issue): 6–16.

Chapter 3

Think globally, act locally
What are the implications for health promotion and research?

Hilary Whent

Introduction

This chapter is based on a study that was carried out in 1996 for the Health Education Authority and in part fulfilment of an M.Sc. in Health Promotion Sciences at the London School of Hygiene and Tropical Medicine. The aims of the study were to explore the features of Agenda 21 and its policy context, to describe and evaluate how Agenda 21 is progressing in Britain with reference to health promotion and to discuss the implications for health promotion and research. Methods used in this study included literature searches, document analysis, in depth interviews with people working on Agenda 21 and observation at meetings.

What is Agenda 21?

Agenda 21 is a far-reaching international environment and development plan that was agreed and signed by the world's heads of state in 1992 at the Earth Summit in Rio de Janeiro. The plan provides a framework for working towards the concept of sustainable development. Sustainable development is the response to the prospect of global ecological breakdown due to planetary overload. For example, based on current estimates of consumption and known reserves, CFCs and similar compounds are damaging the defensive ozone layer. Emissions of gases such as carbon dioxide into the atmosphere contribute to global warming (Crombie 1995, McMichael 1994). While many of the impacts of these changes appear to be most graphically illustrated in the poorer countries, they are by no means confined to tropical regions. Supplies of minerals, such as lead, zinc and mercury, will be exhausted in less than twenty-five years. Marine stocks, topsoil, forests and fresh water are all being consumed faster than they are being replaced.

Although sustainable development has origins in environmental policy, it has emerged as an 'umbrella' concept under which a complex array of interrelated issues can be gathered relating to global crisis. Reid (1995) highlights three main issues: the increase in human-related activities and their impacts and an accompanying decrease in the resources of the planet; growing inequity between rich and poor – between rich and poor nations and between rich and poor within some countries; and population growth.

The term 'sustainable development' first came to prominence in the World Conservation Strategy published by the World Conservation Union in 1980. It has been variously defined but the classic definition comes from the report of the World Commission on Environment and Development *Our Common Future* (or Brundtland Report): 'development that meets the needs of current generations without compromising the ability of future generations to meet their needs' (World Commission on Environment and Development 1987).

The commission was asked by the UN General Assembly to propose long-term environmental strategies for achieving sustainable development by the year 2000 and beyond and to formulate a global agenda for change. In the report it was recognised that to move towards sustainable development required the integration and reconciliation of many different objectives: protection of the natural and cultural environment; improvement of health; tackling poverty, social exclusion and inequality (World Commission on Environment and Development 1987). So, for example, improved air quality may require changes to business development policies, transport policies and town planning.

The Agenda 21 document, which came out of the Earth Summit in 1992, is an action plan for sustainable development. It contains forty chapters with sections on: social and economic development; conservation and management of resources for development; strengthening the role of major groups involved in achieving sustainable development; and means of implementation. The plan makes reference to the roles of international, national and local authorities in achieving sustainable development. A key role in implementing the plan rests with local authorities, which charged with producing a Local Agenda 21 (LA21) plan by 1996. The nature of Agenda 21 is thus well captured by the environmental slogan 'think globally, act locally'. At a local level in Britain, the

Local Government Management Board has described features of a sustainable community (see Figure 3.1).

Community participation in decision-making and action is identified as a crucial part of delivering Agenda 21. This was because the need to construct broadly based consensus approaches was

---

Figure 3.1   Features of a sustainable environment

- Resources are used efficiently, waste is minimised and materials recycled
- Pollution is limited to levels which do not cause damage to natural ecosystems
- The diversity of nature is valued and protected
- Where possible, local needs are met locally
- Everyone has access to adequate food, water, shelter and fuel at a reasonable cost
- Everyone has the opportunity to undertake satisfying work in a diverse economy
- The value of unpaid work is recognised, and payment for work is both fair and fairly distributed
- Health is protected by the creation of safe, clean and pleasant environments and of services which emphasise prevention of illness as well as care for the sick
- Access to facilities, services, goods and other people is not achieved at the expense of the environment or limited to those with cars
- People live without fear of crime, or persecution on account of their race, gender, sexuality or beliefs
- Everyone has access to the skills, knowledge and information which they need to play a full part in society
- All sections of the community are empowered to participate in decision-making
- Opportunities to participate in culture, leisure and recreation are readily available to all
- Buildings, open spaces and artefacts combine meaning with beauty and utility; settlements are 'human' in scale and form and diversity and distinctive local features are valued and protected

Source: Local Government Management Board (1995)

acknowledged and agreed. Chapter 28 of the plan specifically mentions the need to involve different interests and minorities in the processes of preparing each strategy.

What are the links between sustainable development and health promotion?

There are many explicit references to health in Agenda 21. The chapter entitled 'Protecting and promoting human health' covers five programme areas: meeting primary health care needs particularly in rural areas, control of communicable diseases, protecting vulnerable groups, meeting the urban health challenge and reducing health risk from environmental pollution and hazards. The origins of this chapter are in the World Health Organization's (WHO) European Region 'Health For All' targets and related plans and charters, including the Ottawa Charter on Health Promotion. Therefore, the WHO principles that inequalities in health should be addressed, that the determinants of health include physical, socio-economic and cultural environmental factors, that both the development of healthy public policy and the creation of active empowered communities are necessary for creating a health promoting environment (WHO *et al.* 1986) are all encapsulated in the Agenda 21 plan.

Labonte (1991) provides a useful framework for considering the interaction between sustainable development and health. Three relationships are identified in Figure 3.2.

Links between the environment and health are well established. The most fully examined health impacts of the environment are those involving a direct physical or chemical effect – for example waste disposal, air pollution, transport, noise, drinking water and environmental radiation (Crombie 1995, Department of Health/ Department of Environment 1996, WHO 1992). However, there are many, less tangible effects on health and health behaviour linked to the environment, for example facilities for safe play and physical activity and access to healthy foods and opportunities for social development (Crombie 1995, Benzeval *et al.* 1995, Rogers *et al.* 1997). There is also inequality in the distribution of access to healthy environments (MacIntyre and Ellaway 1996).

A country's economic policies, such as how a government chooses to stimulate economic growth, how it deals with balance-of-payments and budgetary deficits, and the control of inflation,

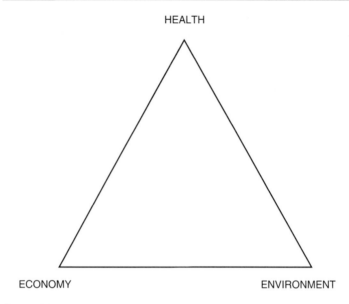

HEALTH

ECONOMY   ENVIRONMENT

Figure 3.2   Sustainable development and health
Source: Labonte (1991)

impact on health in a number of ways. The World Bank (1993) demonstrated that, in global terms, while there is a strong relationship between Gross National Product (GNP) and health measures such as life expectancy, particularly in developing countries, this is not a linear relationship and increased life expectancy tapers off as GNP increases in richer countries. Also, economic progress is assessed mainly by GNP which only counts marketed activities and counts them positively whether they are positive or negative for health. At an individual level poverty and unemployment have negative effects on health (Bartley 1994). At a population level Wilkinson (1996) has shown that industrialised countries with more equitable distributions of income have better health, as for example measured by life expectancy, than those where incomes are more unequally distributed. Economic decisions may also have large effects internationally on health. Crombie (1995) cites debt payments from so-called developing countries to the developed world. Globalisation of the market place means that there is no necessity for profits to be used for the benefit of the area in which they are made.

The environment and the economy are inextricably linked. Conventional economic systems do not take account of environmental costs (i.e. externalities). For example, GNP, which is used as a traditional indicator of economic growth, does not take account of factors such as environmental damage or disintegration of communities.

UK response to Agenda 21

At a national level the UK Government published its response to Rio, *Sustainable Development: The UK Strategy*, in 1994. Three new arrangements were introduced as part of this strategy. The Government Panel on Sustainable Development was set up to advise the Conservative Prime Minister, John Major, on sustainability issues, to monitor progress and to consider priorities. Themes covered in its first report were environmental pricing and economic instruments, environmental education and training, depletion of fish stocks, ozone depletion, reform of the Common Agricultural Policy, climate change, transport, indicators and targets (Department of Environment 1995). A UK Round Table on Sustainable Development was also established, bringing together representatives from private, public and voluntary sectors to build consensus. A national public education initiative called 'Going for Green' was launched to increase public awareness of, and to encourage action on, environmental issues. This campaign includes the promotion of a Green Code: 'cutting down waste, saving energy and natural resources, travelling sensibly, preventing pollution, looking after the local environment'. Five pilot 'sustainable communities' projects were set up with local authorities. These aim to examine the factors which 'encourage or prevent people from adopting environmentally responsible behaviour and also monitor the environmental, social and economic impacts which result from a small community adopting the lifestyle changes promoted by the Green Code'. In each pilot local authority a local management team is being drawn together to secure local involvement. Local universities are being enlisted to provide research and evaluation support. The campaign funds the Eco-schools award, which is an international initiative to help schools combine environmental education with practical measures (personal communication with Marketing Manager, Campaign Pack, Going for Green, 1996).

A critique of the Conservative Government's approach was that environmental issues and economic development were kept separate, rather than being integrated, in the spirit of sustainable development. Wilks and Hall (1995) argued that it was the continuation of an approach which has seen emergent environmental policies co-exist with 'strongly de-regulatory, market-orientated ideology. Emphasis was on voluntary enforcement of environmental good practice rather than legally based regulation' (ibid.) and exhortation of individuals to change their behaviour without the necessary supportive public policy.

A similar approach was adopted with regard to health. References to health in *Sustainable Development: The UK Strategy* only related to specific hazards. The national strategy for health *Health of the Nation*, which was published the same year (Department of Health 1992) as Rio, focused on diseases and their behavioural determinants, placing emphasis on individual action to address these. There was some reference to multi-sectoral collaboration in the form of 'healthy alliances' but again there was a lack of linkage to economic and environmental factors that impact on health.

It is too early to comment on the current UK Government's approach to sustainable development. *Opportunities for Change*, a consultation document, was published in January 1998 and a new public health strategy for England, *Our Healthier Nation* was published for consultation in February 1998. Within these documents and other policy initiatives there is a much clearer articulation of the links between the economy, health and well-being and the environment, together with a commitment to tackle inequalities, and to encourage community participation and move away from placing sole responsibility on individuals for their health and behaviour towards an acknowledgement of the role of the environment.

Local Agenda 21

Local authorities are expected to deliver two-thirds of the Agenda 21 plan, hence the slogan 'think globally, act locally'. Even before the Rio Earth Summit, a number of local government bodies had begun to take on environment and development initiatives, for example setting up Environment Fora involving businesses, community groups and academics, carrying out 'State of the Environment' reporting and a Green Audit. Some local authorities, such as London Borough of Camden and Liverpool City Council, have been participating in the WHO Healthy Cities initiative, set up in 1986, which aims to mobilise local governments and communities to achieving WHO's 'Health for All' strategy and, in principle, links health, environment and social well-being (Ashton and Seymour 1988).

The Local Government Management Board (LGMB) has been at the forefront of providing support and guidance to local authorities on Local Agenda 21 (LA21). A LGMB Survey found that, in 1996, 91 per cent of local authorities claimed commitment to the process and 40 per cent said they had a sustainable development strategy. The Labour Government has set a target that they should all put in place LA21 strategies by the year 2000.

No extra funds have been allocated nationally. It is expected that resources will be made available within local authorities. The majority of authorities have added new duties to the jobs of existing officers and a significant proportion has set up new posts to take this agenda forward.

In practice, local authorities are using a range of management tools as part of LA21. 'State of the Environment' reporting attempts to describe features of the local environment and make an assessment of its quality. Some are using the Eco-Management and Audit Scheme (EMAS) which helps local authorities to set and make progress towards their own chosen targets of environmental performance. A distinction is made between local authorities' direct impact on the environment (for example, paper use, council transport, heating of offices) and service effects (for example, energy efficiency of council housing, disposal of household rubbish). Other local authorities are using sustainability audit, which is an emerging appraisal methodology for reviewing policy or programme options against the many-faceted objectives of sustainable development. 'This means assessing impacts on not only the environment but quality of life for this and future generations' (The Chartered Institute of Environmental Health 1995).

The development of indicators is seen as an important part of the LA21 process, in order to quantify and monitor sustainability performance. LGMB commissioned a Sustainability Indicators research project that aimed to develop and pilot indicators for local authority use. The most commonly used indicators are given in Figure 3.3.

Figure 3.3   Sustainability indicators

- domestic waste production per person per year
- percentage of total domestic waste collection for recycling
- area of open land lost to developments
- local air quality indicators
- percentage of river mileage falling within Class One
- rate of long-term unemployment
- child asthma per 1000
- passenger miles by transport mode per capita

Source: Local Government Management Board (1995)

Education and awareness raising are key features of LA21 work. Training sessions are organised with both local authority employees and elected members and with the public, for example, giving talks in schools, to local businesses and community groups. About half of authorities publish local environmental information such as leaflets on waste disposal and energy use. The majority aim to generate coverage of the initiative in local newspapers and about 20 per cent have some kind of information or resources centre (London Ecology Centre 1995).

Community participation is seen as vital to the LA21 process (Earth Summit 1992). In 1995, 28 per cent of authorities had adapted existing public consultation procedures and a third have set up new mechanisms (London Ecology Centre 1995). A range of methods are being used for example public meetings, question-naires, focus groups, community visioning (Burton 1997). Although few authorities are adopting a truly 'bottom up' approach, LA21 has generated opportunities for traditional non-participants and communities of interest to gain access to decision-making channels (Young 1995). One of the features of the process is to encourage local people to identify projects that they can set up and run themselves. These aim to meet their needs in the informal or social economy on a not-for-profit basis, or would be projects that con-tribute to environmental improvement and enhance quality of life. These consist of activities such as adopting recycling banks, running Local Exchange Trading Systems (LETS), setting up credit unions, urban food growing, community transport schemes, tree warden initiatives, and 'safer routes to school' initiatives that encourage parents to seek alternative ways of taking children to school rather than using the car.

Qualitative research using focus groups, carried out in 1995, into public perceptions of sustainability found that people held positive views about sustainable development once the concept was explained to them and were supportive of some of the notions connected with it. However, lack of trust in central and local government, and anxiety and pessimism about current social trends, such as job insecurity, growth of crime and perceived loss of power of local authorities, was found amongst those who took part in the focus groups. The researchers concluded that these factors will make it difficult to engage many individuals in the LA21 process (Macnaghten *et al.* 1995). A key theme which emerged from interviews with officers working on LA21 was a concern that public expectations will be raised and remain unfulfilled.

The links between health and sustainable development were discussed earlier in the chapter and it is important to consider what happens in practice at the local level. In Britain, responsibility for development and implementation of local health strategies rests with district health authorities. In 1996, there appeared to be little involvement of health authorities in LA21. There may be a number of reasons for this. The political links between local authorities and the NHS are many and complex. Joint planning structures are dominated by community care issues. Some public health or health promotion groups emerged in the 1980s but progress has been slow and patchy. A survey of health promotion work in local authorities in England found evidence of some joint working in terms of specific projects, for example Healthy Cities initiatives, work under the *Health of the Nation* healthy alliance banner and input into each others' strategies and joint funding of posts (HEA/LGMB 1997).

There are significant barriers to collaboration, for example organisational changes, fragmentation in services planning and delivery, and different agendas. The national picture, that conceptually and practically keeps apart issues of health, environment and economics, is largely replicated at a local level. Local authorities traditionally have a role in health in terms of environmental health and their functions, such as housing, planning, social services and education, impact on the determinants of health. Responsibility for public health was with local authorities until 1974 when the Medical Officers for Health transferred to the local NHS. In 1992, lead responsibility for delivering *Health of the Nation* at a local level was given to District Health Authorities with local authorities being encouraged to link with them in 'healthy alliances' (Department of Health 1992). A number of local authorities were critical of *Health of the Nation*, stating that it was too narrowly focused on diseases and neglected socio-economic and environmental determinants of health and the contribution that local government made to these (various, personal communication; Blackman 1995).

The Labour Government has articulated the concept of sustainable development within its recently published consultative policy documents. Local authorities have been given a new statutory duty to promote the economic, social and environmental well-being of their area, working with local people, businesses and voluntary organisations. *Our Healthier Nation* makes links with LA21 and it is stated that Health Improvement Programmes will provide a central vehicle for advancing local health within each health authority's region, including locally determined priorities and targets. The lead role for this will be health authorities but in partnership with local authorities and other organisations (Department of Health 1998).

Given concern that the focus of LA21 activities tends to be dominated by 'green/environment' issues without encapsulating the concept of sustainable development (London Ecology Centre 1996), it has been suggested that those involved in the LA21 process could benefit from a health promotion perspective and 'health' in its fullest sense should be emphasised in the ongoing discourse of sustainable development (Young 1995, Rogers and Whyms 1995, Labonte 1991, Brown *et al.*1992). As an example, Young presents the case of town planners. He argues that a fuller understanding of the health implications of policies would help planners to develop more holistic approaches to policy-making; they could learn about environmental education and in the promotion of participation from those involved in community development approaches in health promotion (Young 1995). In practice, much of LA21 work is informational and concerned with encouraging behaviour change with regards to the environment. The wealth of findings from health promotion research into lifestyles could usefully be disseminated to this audience.

In practice, health promotion work has tended to involve individualistic approaches to encouraging behaviour change (Gillies 1998). The Agenda 21 initiative offers the opportunity to take a more broad-based approach to promoting health within the concept of sustainable development. As discussed above, there are signs of increased recognition of Agenda 21 and its opportunities for promoting public health within government policy and amongst the public health community. Sustainable development and health has been a key theme discussed at national public health conferences. For example, in 1997 the Association for Public Health conference focused on the environment and health, and in 1996 the Public Health Alliance's Annual General Meeting discussed 'Greening Health'. Several national alliances have set up projects which disseminate examples of practice which link up health to sustainable development within communities. For example, the Public Health Alliance has begun producing a resource pack on sustainable development and health; and the National Food Alliance has set up a project which looks at the potential of urban food growing to form a practical tangible link between health, the environment and a cohesive community (Garnett 1996). Examples of local projects which link sustainable development and health are noted below:

- A private company 'Heatwise' in Glasgow acts to improve people's environment and health while tackling unemployment. It provides training for formerly unemployed people and carries out work to rehabilitate cold, damp houses. Funds are provided from earned income, district councils and the European Social Fund. This results in energy efficiency measures, fuel cost savings, improved health status of inhabitants, and employment opportunities for those trained (Public Health Alliance 1995).
- The Soil Association has set up a Local Food Links (offering advice to LA21 partnerships) initiative, which aims to market local agricultural or horticultural produce to local consumers. The scheme is suitable for small business, consumers get fresh food of high nutritional value. Other benefits are an increase in the viability of small farms, the creation of local employment and the encouragement of healthy eating. As part of LA21, a partnership between the project, Devon County Council, Ministry of Agriculture Food and Fisheries and Plymouth and Torbay Health Authority is working to establish one of these links (Bridger and Morgan 1996).
- Lancashire County Council's LA21 action plan identified cycling as an activity to be encouraged and promoted by: examining the potential for transferring journeys from car to bicycle, and setting targets to meet this potential; segregated cycle networks;

traffic calming to equalise vehicle and cycle speeds; secure, conveniently located parking and storage facilities for cycles; varying cycle parking standards applied to new developments according to the identified potential and needs of cyclists (Lancashire County Council 1993).

Health promotion research and LA21

There is an urgent need to find ways of linking up the numerous health related strategies in order that resources can be channelled appropriately and not duplicated, and that local people are not over-consulted and exhorted to participate in different sectors initiatives which they see as related.

A number of recommendations can be made for health promotion research. This study highlights the need to carry out more policy analysis. This discipline uses a range of mainly qualitative research techniques, such as interviews, focus groups, document analysis and political mapping. Given that the determinants of health are affected by a whole range of policies and agencies, we need such research which is 'not only concerned with the process of policy-making but that is concerned with the behaviour of actors in formulating and implementing policy and the context within which policies are promulgated' (Walt and Gilson 1994). This research will help those seeking to promote health identify opportunities for influencing the policy process and policy actors.

Health promotion research should contribute to the development of sustainability audits by exploring how health could be taken into account. In Britain, the health sector is currently developing methodologies for carrying out health impact assessments; this work should link with Agenda 21 work. However, a key issue is whether the findings from such assessments are incorporated into decision-making.

There is also a need to develop measures of success for initiatives which aim to make progress towards health and sustainable development. Health promotion research could investigate what health indicators are worth looking at in relation to sustainable development. Some of these indicators would have to be developed through participatory work with communities but some would have to be correlated with major health concerns such as low birth weight, mental well-being, coronary heart disease. Research currently being carried out to investigate the links between social capital and health and the development of social indicators for health promotion at a community level may help to inform this work (Gillies 1998, Cooper *et al.* 1999). Social capital refers to the cohesion that results when a community is characterised by a rich associational life. Putnam, a political scientist, defines social capital in terms of a number of community characteristics 'the existence of community networks, civic engagement, civic identity, reciprocity and trust of others in the community' (Putnam 1995). There is evidence that the extent of social capital in a community is likely to affect health (Kawachi *et al.* 1996, Kawachi *et al.* 1997, Wilkinson 1996). An international review of approaches to improving health through community partnerships found that the recurring themes of good social relationships, social and civic activities (all relevant to Agenda 21 work) were seen to be fundamental to influencing the health behaviour of individuals, the health status of populations and the broader social and environmental contexts of health (Gillies 1998).

Agenda 21 was heralded as a ground-breaking document, providing an action plan for working towards sustainable development. Sustainable development and health promotion policy intersect in many ways. An analysis of progress in Britain indicates that Agenda 21 work could be enhanced with a health promotion perspective and that the initiative provides an opportunity to promote public health.

References

Ashton J., Seymour H. (1988) *The New Public Health. The Liverpool Experience*. Milton Keynes: Open University Press.

Bartley M. (1994) 'Unemployment and ill health: understanding the relationship'. *Journal of Epidemiology and Community Health* 48: 333–7.

Benzeval M., Judge K., Whitehead M. (eds) (1995) *Tackling Inequalities in Health: An Agenda for Action*. London: Kings Fund.

Blackman T. (1995) 'Recent developments in British national health policy: an emerging role for local government'. *Policy and Politics* 23: 31–48.

Bridger R., Morgan D. (1996) 'Food and land links'. *Sustainable London*: 15.

Brown V. *et al.* (1992) 'Health promotion and environmental management: a partnership for the future'. *Health Promotion International* 7: 219–30.

Burton P. (1997) *Community Visioning: An Evaluation of the 'Choices for Bristol' Project*. Bristol: The Policy Press.

The Chartered Institute of Environmental Health (1995) *Environmental Health for Sustainable Development. An Illustrated Guide by the Chartered Institute of Environmental Health*. CIOEH.

Cooper H., Arber S., Ginn J. (1999). *The Influence of Social Support and Social Capital on Health. A Review and Analysis of British Data*. London: Health Education Authority.

Crombie H. (1995) *Sustainable Development and Health, A Public Health Trust Project*. Public Health Alliance.

Department of Environment (1995) *British Government Panel on Sustainable Development, First Report*. London: Department of Environment.

Department of Health (1992) *The Health of the Nation: A Strategy for Health in England*. London: HMSO.

—— (1998) *Our Healthier Nation*. London: HMSO.

Department of Health/Department of the Environment (1996) *UK Environmental Health Action Plan*. London: HMSO.

Earth Summit '92 (1992) *The United Nations Conference on Environment and Development*. Rio de Janeiro: The Regency Press.

Garnett T. (1996) In: London Ecology Centre *Linking up London for a Sustainable Future*. Conference report. London: London Ecology Centre.

Gillies P. (1998) 'Effectiveness of alliances and partnerships for health promotion'. *Health Promotion International* 13: 99–119.

Health Education Authority/Local Government Management Board (1997) *Promoting Health in Local Government*. London: Health Education Authority.

Kawachi I., Colditz G., Asherio A., Rimm E., Giovannucci E., Stampger M., Willett W. (1996) 'A prospective study of social networks in relation to total mortality and cardiovascular disease in men in the USA'. *Journal of Epidemiology and Community Health* 50: 245–51.

Kawachi I., Kennedy B., Lochner K., Prothrew-Stith D. (1997) 'Social capital, income inequality and mortality'. *American Journal of Public Health* 89: 491–8.

Lancashire County Council (1993) *Lancashire Environment Action Programme: A Local Agenda 21 for Lancashire*.

Labonte R. (1991) 'Econology: integrating health and sustainable development. Part One: theory and background'. *Health Promotion International* 6: 49–65.

Local Government Management Board (1995) *Indicators for Local Agenda 21 – A Summary. Sustainability Indicators Research Project*.

London Ecology Centre (1995) *Progress of the 33 London Boroughs on Local Agenda 21*. London Ecology Centre in association with the Association of London Government, Local Government Management Board and the London Ecology Unit.

—— (1995/96). *Sustainable London*. The Quarterly Newsletter of the London Agenda 21 Network.

MacIntyre S., Ellaway A. (1996) 'Social and Local variation in the use of urban neighbourhoods: a case study in Glasgow', unpublished mimeo. Glasgow: Medical Research Council

Macnaghten P. *et al.* (1995) *Public Perceptions and Sustainability in Lancashire: Indicators, Institutions, Participation. A Report by the Centre for the Study of Environmental Change Commissioned by Lancashire Country Council.* Lancaster: Lancaster University Centre for the Study of Environmental Change.

McMichael A. (1994) *Planetary Overload.* Cambridge: Cambridge University Press.

Public Health Alliance (1995) 'Public Health Alliance sustainable development and health project'. *Community Health Action* 35: 9.

Putnam R. (1995) 'Tuning in, tuning out: the strange disappearance of social capital'. *American Political Science and Politics*: 664–83.

Reid D. (1995) *Sustainable Development: An Introductory Guide.* London: Earthscan.

Rogers A., Popay J., Williams G. (1997) *Inequalities in Health and Health Promotion: Insights from the Qualitative Research Literature.* London: Health Education Authority.

Rogers A., Whyms D. (1995) 'Health and ecology'. *Health Matters* 2: 12–13.

Walt G., Gilson G. (1994) 'Reforming the health sector in developing countries: the central role of policy analysis'. *Health Policy and Planning* 9: 353–370.

Wilkinson R. (1996) *Unhealthy Societies. The Afflictions of Inequality.* London: Routledge.

Wilks S., Hall P. (1995) 'Think globally, act locally: implementing Agenda 21 in Britain'. *Policy Studies* 16: 37–44.

World Bank (1993) *World Development Report 1993: Investing in Health.* New York: Oxford University Press.

World Commission on Environment and Development (1987) *Our Common Future* (The Brundtland Report). Oxford: Oxford University Press.

World Health Organization (1992) *Our Planet, our Health. Report of the WHO Commission on Health and Environment.* Geneva: World Health Organization.

—— (1986) *Ottawa Charter for Health Promotion. An International Conference on Health Promotion.* Copenhagen: World Health Organization, Regional Office for Europe.

Young S. (1995) 'Participation – out with the old, in with the new'. *Town and Country Planning* 64: 110–12.

Chapter 4

A critical approach to lifestyle and health

Thomas Abel, William C. Cockerham and Steffen Niemann

Introduction

Lifestyle has become a popular concept, not just in the social and health sciences, but in Western societies at large. In market economies lifestyle signifies important consumer groups and in politics, lifestyle is frequently referred to in rhetorics that emphasise individual over social responsibility. In the social sciences the lifestyle approach is traditionally used as a secondary concept in the debate on the relative importance of social conditions and behaviours for social inequalities. More recently in sociology, the term lifestyle is prominently applied to describe new forms of social differentiation under post-modern or high modernity conditions (e.g. Giddens 1991, Featherstone 1991). And, finally, lifestyle as an 'in vogue' term in the health sciences, is unfortunately often misused either as an empty phrase applied to sell the research community old ideas under a new heading or as a hotchpotch category for almost everything that somehow has to do with social behaviour and health.

In medical sociology the lifestyle idea is frequently employed in the polarised debate about materialist or behavioural explanations of health inequalities. As Macintyre (1997) observes, one of the major problems in this debate is that it has diverted attention from the bigger questions about the precise mechanisms or pathways by which social inequalities in health are generated and maintained in particular contexts.

This chapter attempts to show that important insights into the complex relationship between social and health inequality can be obtained by applying a theory-based sociological approach to lifestyles. It will demonstrate that a first and fundamental task for health lifestyle research today is to be more precise in the terminology, particularly the use of the term lifestyle. And finally, new directions for the development of more comprehensive empirical models of health related lifestyles will be outlined.

Earlier lifestyle approaches in health research

The growing interest in the associations between lifestyle and health goes back about thirty years to the early studies in the USA (e.g. 'Alameda County', 'Framingham'). The major contribution of these studies was the identification of particular behaviours that significantly effect mortality and morbidity, especially behavioural risk factors such as smoking, excessive alcohol consumption, physical inactivity and overweight (e.g. Berkman and Breslow 1983, Castelli and Anderson 1986). Consequently, similar studies were conducted in Europe, for example the North Karelia Study from Scandinavia (Puska *et al.* 1995) and the multi-national MONICA Project (WHO MONICA Project Principal Investigators 1988), and in many other parts of the world. However, such earlier studies were basically exploratory and descriptive and most lacked a theoretical basis. There are five points of critique that are of major importance here.

First, a focus on a single health behaviour does not adequately represent the complexity of behavioural effects on health. The development of risk behaviours, as well as their specific effects on health, need to be studied on the basis of their interrelated patterns and complex interactions. In that sense using additive indices that sum single health behaviours (Harris and Guten 1979, Mechanic and Cleary 1980) into a cumulative score does not present an appropriate method. Cumulative measures tend to disguise differentiated effects, such as inconsistency in patterns of health behaviours or interaction effects between single health behaviours (e.g. Abel *et al.* 1992).

Second, a focus on risk or health damaging behaviours is restrictive, since it neglects the complexity typical of processes of health maintenance or health risk. For a more comprehensive understanding of the relationship between health and lifestyle, health protective and health promoting factors need to be given more attention (e.g. Noack 1988).

Third, a perspective that concentrates on individuals tends to overlook social structural and group specific effects on health behaviour. It neglects the fact that development and maintenance of health behaviour is strongly influenced by the structural, social and group specific context of the actor (Bandura 1985, Siegrist 1995). A perspective focused on the individual does not provide for a comprehensive understanding of such processes.

Fourth, with increasing knowledge about the importance of social and cultural contexts, exclusive concentration on behavioural aspects of lifestyles becomes problematic. The study of the relationship between lifestyle and health requires more comprehensive lifestyle models that incorporate cultural, social and psychological effects.

Finally, in most previous studies a specification of the associations among health lifestyle factors is missing. The majority shows a concentration on bivariate dependency links, while interdependencies and recursive associations are often neglected (Dean 1993). Yet, complexity of conditions and effect patterns among specific lifestyle factors is a core element of the health lifestyle approach. Thus, perhaps the major weakness in these earlier studies was their neglect of the complexities linking distinct behaviours and between the behaviours and their biopsychosocial correlates. The most basic question appears unanswered: 'How can we measure health lifestyles without reducing their complexities to a degree that it is no longer lifestyles but rather risk behaviours that we study?' From the empirical perspective, this question points to the perhaps most crucial and challenging, yet unresolved, issue in lifestyle research to date.

While many so-called lifestyle studies today still follow the epidemiological risk factor paradigm, a few recent studies have made attempts to overcome some of the restriction of the earlier approaches. Perhaps most prominent among them is the *Health and Lifestyle Survey* by Mildred Blaxter and her colleagues (Blaxter 1990). The aim of this study was to analyse the relationships between attitudes, circumstances, behaviours and health. Thus, their study applied a significantly wider scope than most epidemiological studies. Taking a sociological perspective, a major focus in the Blaxter study was on issues of social inequality and health. The results confirmed earlier findings of the effect of social circumstances on health and health behaviours. Health was significantly related to social class, housing tenure, single parent status, social integration and other social determinants. Health was also related to various behaviour patterns such as smoking, exercise and diet. Health behaviours in turn were associated with social class, for example, smoking with education and exercise with occupational class.

Blaxter's work is primarily concerned with health as the outcome variable. With respect to the sociological issue of inequality, it starts by taking an 'either–or' perspective that examines social circumstances in contrast to behavioural effects on health. Yet, in the final chapter, an attempt is made to study the joint effect of social circumstances and behaviours on health. It is in this later part that the Blaxter study has drawn the most attention outside Britain. Approaching issues of interactions of behavioural and structural determinants on health, Blaxter finds preliminary support that health promoting effects of certain behaviours depend on social class related circumstances. 'If circumstances are good, healthy behaviour appears to have a strong influence upon health. If they are bad, then behaviours make rather little difference' (Blaxter 1990).

The empirical evidence for an interdependency of structural and behavioural effects on health is perhaps the most stimulating finding from Blaxter's study. Although consecutive research has raised some doubt about the cross-national validity of this finding (Kooiker and Christiansen 1995), this part of Blaxter's study points to new directions in health research. In particular, it highlights the need to explore issues of complex interaction among structural and behavioural determinants of health. However, as Blaxter's work is predominantly concerned with health as an outcome, rather little attention is given to the definition of her concept of lifestyle. She applies a wide definition that is basically focused on behaviours, either voluntarily chosen or more or less influenced by economic or cultural conditions. Her primary interest in lifestyles appears to be its use as a concept which is antagonistic to the social determination of health.

The main thesis of the present chapter is that the lifestyle approach has more to offer than serving as a synonym for patterns of risk behaviours or as a vaguely defined concept to describe in a more general form the behavioural aspect in health. We try to show that using a theory driven lifestyle approach can help not only to prevent a reductionist and individual centred perspective, but that the lifestyle approach supports a better understanding of the interplay of social circumstances and behaviours. In fact, it will be argued that linking social structural and behavioural aspects presents the real and genuine contribution of the lifestyle approach in the health sciences.

Health related lifestyles and social differentiation: from theory to empirical concepts

As soon as we start thinking about a definition of lifestyle or search for particular lifestyle indicators, we immediately recognise the need for theoretical criteria or guidance. Without those, lifestyle could refer to merely everything that relates to people's lives which would, however, render the lifestyle approach useless in social and health sciences.

Fortunately, a number of leading sociologists have incorporated lifestyle in their theories. We find definitions and explanations of lifestyle in classical sociological theories such as in the work of Georg Simmel and, from contemporary theorists, for example Anthony Giddens (see Cockerham *et al.* 1993).

Max Weber[1]

Among the classical theorists, Max Weber provided the deepest insight into the lifestyle concept and the foundation for subsequent lifestyle research (Wrong 1990). Weber (1978: 932) linked lifestyles to status by pointing out that a distinguishing characteristic of status is 'status honour' or prestige which is normally expressed by the fact that above all else a specific style of life is expected from all those who wish to belong to the circle. Status, not class, plays the larger role in Weber's perspective. Weber views class strictly as a reflection of the marketplace, signifying a person's level of income, property, or economic skill. Status groups, on the other hand, are aggregates of people with similar status, class backgrounds and political influence, and they originate through a sharing of similar lifestyles or as a means to preserve a particular style of life. Weber observed that lifestyles were based not so much on what a person produced, but on what he or she consumed. As Weber (1978: 933) put it: 'one might thus say that classes are stratified according to their relations to the production and acquisition of goods; whereas status groups are stratified according to the principles of their consumption of goods as represented by special styles of life'.

Consumption is, of course, not independent of production; rather, lifestyle differences between status groups are based on their relationship to the means of consumption, not the means of production. The economic mode of production sets the basic parameters within which consumption occurs, but does not deter-mine or even necessarily affect specific forms of it (Bocock 1993). This is because the consumption of goods and services conveys a social meaning which displays, at the time, the status and social identity of the consumer. Consumption can therefore be regarded as a set of social and cultural practices that establish differences between social groups, not merely means of expressing differences which are already in place because of economic factors (ibid.: 64, Bourdieu 1984). It is the use of particular goods and services through distinct lifestyles that ultimately distinguishes status groups from one another.

Three terms in the original German are used by Weber to express his concept of lifestyles. These terms are Stilisierung des Lebens (stylisation of life) or, more simply, Lebensstil (lifestyle), along with Lebensführung (life conduct), and Lebenschancen (life chances) which make up the two sides of lifestyles (Abel and Cockerham 1993, Cockerham *et al.* 1993) (see Figure 4.1). Lebensführung refers to the choices that people have in their selection of lifestyles and Lebenschancen is the probability of realising those choices.

This major distinction in Weber's concept of lifestyles has been obscured in English language translations of his *Wirtschaft und Gesellschaft* (Abel and Cockerham 1993). In Gerth and Mills (Weber 1946) and Roth and Wittch (Weber 1978), the most freq-uently cited English versions, 'Stilisierung des Lebens' and 'Lebensführung' are both mutually translated as 'lifestyles'. Yet, 'Lebensführung', translated literally, means life conduct and refers to choice or self-direction in behaviour, not lifestyles.

Weber believed that choice is the major factor in the operational-isation of a lifestyle; however, the actualisation of choices is influenced by life chances. Dahrendorf (1979: 73) notes that while

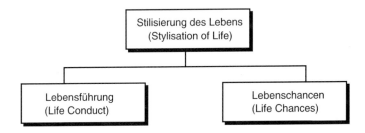

Figure 4.1   Weber on lifestyle

Weber is vague about what he means by life chances, a reasonable definition would be: 'the crystallised probability of finding satisfaction for interests, wants and needs, thus the probability of the occurrence of events which bring about satisfaction'. The probability of acquiring satisfaction is anchored in structural conditions which are largely economic – involving income, property, the opportunity for profit and the like – but Dahrendorf suggests the concept of life chances also involves rights, norms and social relationships (the probability that others will respond in a certain manner). Weber does not consider life chances to be a matter of pure chance; rather, they are the chances people have in life because of their social situation. The overall thesis is that chance is socially determined and social structure is an arrangement of chances. Hence, lifestyles are not random behaviours unrelated to structure, but typically are deliberate choices influenced by life chances.

Consequently, Weber's most important contribution to conceptualising lifestyles in sociological terms is to impose a dialectical capstone over the interplay of choice and structure in lifestyle determination. Choices and constraints work off of one another to determine a distinctive lifestyle for individuals and groups. People have needs, goals, identities and desires, which they match against their chances and probabilities of acquiring them; they then select a lifestyle based on their assessments and the reality of their circumstances. Unrealistic choices are not likely to be achieved or maintained. Realistic choices are based on what is (structurally) possible and are more likely to be operationalised, made routine and can be changed when circumstance permits.

The identification of life chances as the dialectic opposite of choice in Weber's lifestyle scheme provides the theoretical key to understanding how lifestyles are operationalised in the empirical world. It can be said that individuals have a range of freedom, yet not complete freedom, in choosing a lifestyle. That is, people are not entirely free in determining their lifestyle but have the freedom to choose within the social constraints that apply to their situation in life. Lifestyle constraints, in a Weberian context, are primarily socio-economic in origin. Therefore, the value of Weber's concept is that it can account for the interplay of individual choice and structural constraints in operationalising a lifestyle. Those who have the desire and the means may choose; those lacking in some way cannot choose so easily and can find their lifestyle determined more by external circumstances.

Weber's overall contribution to our understanding of contemporary lifestyles is that lifestyles are (1) associated with status groups, therefore they are principally collective, rather than individual, phenomena; (2) lifestyles represent patterns of consumption, not production; and (3) lifestyles are formed by the dialectical interplay between life choices and life chances, with choice playing the greater role. However, in order to understand how life chances determine life choices in contemporary society, it is helpful to turn to more recent sociological theories. In particular Bourdieu's work on social *Distinctions* (1984) provides significant insights.

Pierre Bourdieu

Bourdieu's principal focus is on the question of how routine practices of individuals are influenced by the external structure of their social world and how these practices, in turn, contribute to the maintenance of that structure (Jenkins 1992). This question underlies the basis for Bourdieu's (1990: 53) concept of 'habitus', which he defines as:

> systems of durable, transposable dispositions, structured structures predisposed to operate as structuring structures, that is, as principles which generate and organise practices and representations that can be objectively adapted to their outcomes without presupposing a conscious aiming at ends or an express mastery of the operations necessary in order to attain them.

In other words, knowledge of social structures and conditions produce enduring orientations toward actions that are more or less routine and, when these orientations are acted upon, they tend to reproduce the structures from which they are derived. For example, class culture may influence food habits and these habits collectively help reproduce class culture.

Habitus provides a cognitive map of an individual's social world and the dispositions or 'procedures to follow' appropriate for that person in a particular situation. As Bourdieu explains, the human mind is socially bounded and constructed within the limits of experience, upbringing and training (Bourdieu and Wacquant 1992). People are able to figure out their circumstances, but their perceptions are typically shaped by their social and economic conditions.

> The habitus ... ensures the active presence of past experiences, which, deposited in each organism in the form of schemes of perception, thought and action, tend to guarantee the 'correctness' of practices and their constancy over time, more reliably than all formal rules and explicit norms.
>
> Bourdieu (1990: 54)

Therefore, habitus channels behaviour down paths that appear reasonable to the individual. What this implies for our understanding of lifestyles is the strong influence of structure (i.e. life chances) on the habitus mind-set from which lifestyle choices are derived. This suggests that the selection of, and participation in, a particular lifestyle is affected by life chances to a much greater extent than allowed by Weber. Bourdieu's work indicates that lifestyle choices are not only constrained but shaped by life chances.

Bourdieu (1984: 171) describes the operationalisation of lifestyles as follows: (1) objective conditions of existence combine with positions in the social structure to (2) produce the habitus, which consists of (3) a system of schemes generating classifiable practices and works, and (4) a system of schemes of perception and appreciation (taste) that, together, produce (5) specific classifiable practices and works which (6) result in a lifestyle. Although individuals choose their lifestyles, they do not do so with complete free will, as habitus predisposes them toward certain choices. They have the option to reject or modify these choices, but Bourdieu suggests that an agent's choices are consistent with their habitus. Choices also tend to reflect class position because persons in the same social class share the same habitus. It can, therefore, be argued that structure is the dominant aspect of Bourdieu's concept of lifestyles. The notion of 'structure' suggests persistence, repetition and self-maintenance, hence, habituation. Lifestyles not only reflect social differences in ways of living, but reproduce them.

In sum, Bourdieu's major contribution to our understanding of lifestyles falls into two major areas: first, identifying the role of habitus in creating and reproducing lifestyles; and, second, emphasising this role by going beyond Weber to show how structure, or in Weberian terms, life chances determine lifestyle choices. In Bourdieu's work, the gap between life chances and life choices in Weber's original analysis is significantly reduced through his concept of habitus which incorporates both into a single entity.

Health related lifestyles: a new concept

On the basis of these theoretical accounts we have developed a new approach to health and lifestyles. In our approach we apply a Weberian concept based on the dialectical interplay of life chances and life choices. This dialectic is depicted in Figure 4.2. Recognising the multi-dimensional structure of lifestyles we propose for health related lifestyles the following definition: *health lifestyles comprise interacting patterns of health related behaviours, orientations and resources adapted by groups of individuals in response to their social, cultural and economic environment.*

This definition of health related lifestyles shows particular characteristics. First, it does not limit its scope to the behavioural aspects of lifestyle. It includes individual and structural factors without presupposing strict determinism between such factors. Second, the definition allows us to include perspectives on health held by scientists and lay people. In other words, the selection of behaviours, orientations and resources qualifying as health relevant can be drawn from scientific and lay knowledge. Third, intention is not required in this definition. Health related lifestyles can either be purposefully chosen by individuals for health reasons or they can be rather habitual. However, if intention were to be considered an indispensable feature of a distinct lifestyle, we would suggest defining such lifestyles that are chosen by the individual explicitly for their health effects as health *oriented* lifestyles.

Figure 4.3 displays, in hypothetical form, a possible pattern of health related behaviours, orientations and resources that together form a health related lifestyle. As indicated above, the selection of

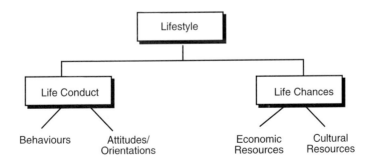

Figure 4.2   Lifestyle, life chances, life conduct

lifestyle elements within each dimension depends on the research questions and may vary greatly while the basic three-dimensional structure persists (Abel 1991).

One of the central issues in this model of health related lifestyle is the nature of the relationships between its dimensions. Here we refer back to Bourdieu's theory on the habitus. Habitus can be seen as a linking mechanism or process that structures the interplay among the lifestyle elements within and between the three constituent dimensions. The habitus shapes the choices people make. It has a continuous effect on everyday actions, perceptions etc. While the habitus shapes people's choices, life chances set the limits within which individuals have more or less options and freedom to choose. Interdependency as a connecting mechanism between life chances and life conduct might be illustrated in an analogy.

The two donkeys in Figure 4.4 indicate the reciprocal relationship between the lifestyle dimensions behaviours and resources. As long as behaviours and resources are in accordance and close to each other (upper part of Figure 4.4) there is conditional freedom for the individual to choose. The habitus as a stirring or regulating mechanism is always present, as here illustrated by the rubber band around the feet of the donkeys. If the two lifestyle dimensions drift apart, however, a confinement factor will increasingly become

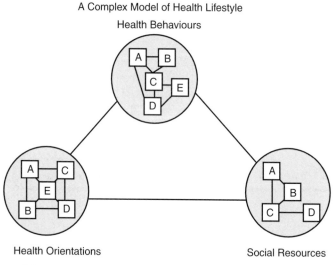

Figure 4.3   Health lifestyle

effective (lower part of Figure 4.4) and the habitus will ensure a readjustment to bring behaviours and resources back into concordance again.

In this analogy, life chances would, like a fence, set the borders or limits for the (re-) adjustment process. These chances are unequally distributed among the social classes, genders, ethnic groups, etc. In line with our theoretical propositions introduced above, life chances set the basic parameters under which most individuals are able to arrange their behaviours and orientations according to their own resources. How to be successful in this task is socially learned *via* the habitus. In this understanding of the relationships between structural and behavioural factors of health, the lifestyle approach leads to new kinds of research questions, for instance: Are health related lifestyles more or less constrained by life chances than other lifestyles? What are the lifestyle restrictions typical for different social status groups, genders etc? What are the central individual enabling factors and the most important structural pre-conditions for the realisation of health promoting lifestyles?

These are basically empirical question for which we have just begun to develop appropriate methods of data collection and analysis. In fact, other more basic empirical issues need to be

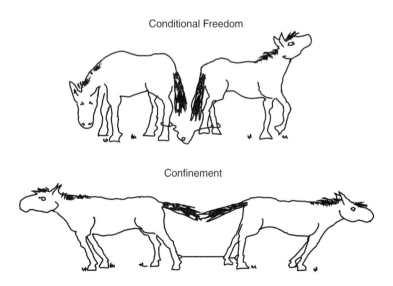

Figure 4.4   Donkey analogy

approached first. For instance, can health related lifestyles, as defined here, be empirically observed in the real world? Can we find evidence for the proposed associations among single health lifestyle elements, and between the three dimensions?

The structure of health related lifestyles: empirical findings

The search for meaningful associations of health lifestyle elements can start at a lower level of complexity by studying bivariate associations between selected behaviours, orientations and resources. Many earlier studies have produced findings that relate to this task. For instance, there is considerable evidence that smoking is associated with education, unemployment and other social determinants. Health relevant orientations such as health locus of control or body perception are also found to correlate significantly with occupational class (e.g. Hayes and Ross 1987, Cockerham *et al.* 1986). Individual resources for health, such as social support or health knowledge, vary by social factors such as gender or social class (e.g. Haug and Lavin 1981, Berkman 1995).

Thus, evidence for meaningful associations between lifestyle elements from all three dimensions is considerable. Yet, it is rather scattered, as most of these findings are not linked to each other in a theoretically meaningful way. This holds true for many other results from earlier studies indicating that health behaviours are linked to each other. Although respective earlier studies may have not used a health lifestyle approach, their results can be linked systematically to the multi-dimensional lifestyle concept. Their findings generally support the idea that individual health behaviours are not independent of each other, that they emerge in larger patterns, and that such patterns are collective phenomena in the sense that they are closely linked to social class, gender and age (Abel and Kohlmann 1989, Uitenbroek 1993, Kickbusch 1986, McQueen 1987).

Most commonly, statistical analyses of the links between lifestyle elements (e.g. health behaviours) and their correlates (e.g. health attitudes) employ causal models such as multiple or logistic regression. However, regression methods basically assume a deterministic link between a dependent variable and a set of explanatory variables. According to our theoretical propositions the links between lifestyle dimensions are, however, rather complex allowing for reciprocity and interaction. Consequently, we need to advance our methods to include the resources directly into statistical models without pre-supposing a strictly deterministic relationship.

Patterns of behaviours and orientations in the health lifestyle perspective: the Bern–Munich lifestyle panel

The Bern–Munich Lifestyle Panel (BMLP) is a longitudinal study that explores structures and dynamics of health related lifestyles among some 2,000 adults in Switzerland and Germany. Its theoretical framework is outlined above. The major tasks of the project are to identify the basic dimensions of health related lifestyles and to study the complex links between structural and behavioural lifestyle elements. Residents of Bern (Switzerland) and Munich (Germany) between the ages of fifty-five and sixty-five years were contacted in twelve-month periods and interviewed by telephone (CATI). Interviews were conducted in two waves in Munich (1996 and 1997) and three waves in Bern (1996/97/98). The questionnaire comprised some two hundred questions on selected aspects of health lifestyles and health status. First descriptive results are published elsewhere (Abel *et al.* 1999). For the present analyses, data from the Swiss part of our study were used.

To explore the relationships between life chances and health related aspects of life conduct we specifically examined the links between social deprivation and selected health orientations and behaviours. With respect to health orientations the BMLP introduces a new measure that was developed to observe people's normative understanding of health behaviours. Health orientations are considered here as a particular form of rational thought and as major determinants of particular health lifestyles. Orientations towards health and health behaviour are based on people's perception of what is and what can realistically be expected with regard to their own health and health behaviour in general. In understanding the forms of rational thought that underlie individual and collective participation in health lifestyles, it is once again useful to employ a Weberian concept. Weber distinguished between two major types of rationality: formal ('Zweckrationalität') and substantive ('Wertrationalität'). Formal rationality is the purposeful calculation of the most efficient means and procedures to realise goals, while substantive rationality is the realisation of values and ideals based on tradition, custom, piety or personal devotion. In Western society, formal rationality was dominant over its substantive counterpart as people sought to achieve certain ends by employing the most efficient means and, in the process, tended to disregard substantive rationality because it often was cumbersome, unnecessarily time-consuming, inefficient and could stifle change. When Weber's concept is applied to health lifestyles, formal rationality appears to be dominant as well. That is, the existing studies show that people do not participate in health lifestyles because health is an idealised end state: rather, they pursue such lifestyles because they want to be healthy in order to use their health as a means to reach chosen goals (d'Houtaud and Field 1984, Cockerham 1998). Health lifestyles are used for the purpose of living longer, avoiding disease, and feeling and looking good. Health lifestyles are therefore chosen largely for practical or utilitarian, not abstract, reasons and valued because they have a practical function to perform.

The BMLP provides the first attempt to apply the theoretically induced categories of formal and substantive rationality to issues of health and behaviour and to operationalise this Weberian concept in an empirical study. Survey questions were developed that asked respondent's normative ideas on why people should engage in health enhancing behaviours and avoid potentially health damaging behaviours. In the BMLP questionnaire an original list of nine items comprised five items that measure formal rationality, such as 'One should behave healthily, because it improves one's own well-being', and four items indicating substantive thoughts, such as 'People should avoid unhealthy behaviour, because it is against nature'. In an earlier analysis of the BMLP data we found preliminary support that formal, but not substantive, rationality orientations were significantly related to health promoting behaviours, in this case participation in sport and physical activity (Abel et al. 1998).

The concept of relative deprivation (Townsend 1979) is applied in the BMLP to study the associations between life chances and behavioural aspects of health. An index of relative deprivation was constructed that measures lack of structural and individual resources. This measure comprises five variables: education, income, housing conditions, leisure time and social support (see Table 4.1).

Using data from the first wave, we applied correspondence analysis to explore the relationships between health related behaviours and orientations and social structural factors. Correspondence analysis is not yet widely used in the Anglo-Saxon social sciences. In French-speaking empirical research, however, it has ranked for

Table 4.1   List of indicators

Variable	Coding
Deprivation Index	Sumscore of five trichotomised resources. Recoded in five categories ranging from low deprivation (Depr− −) to high deprivation (Depr+ +)
Education (highest educational degree)	0 = high degree, 1 = medium degree, 2 = low degree
Income (equivalent income per person in Swiss Francs)	2 = up to 1,800, 1 = 1,801–2,400, 0 = more than 2,400
Living conditions (no. of rooms per person*)	2 = up to 1 room per person, 1 = 1 – 1.5 rooms per person, 0 = more than 1.5 rooms per person
Leisure time (hours of leisure time in a normal working day)	2 = no leisure time, 1 = up to 2 hours leisure time, 0 = more than 2 hours leisure time
Social support (support persons within family)	2 = none, 1 = 1 or 2 persons, 0 = more than 2 persons
Health behaviour	
Sport intensity	Sport− = no sport; Sport+ −= moderate activities; Sport+ = strenuous activities
Cigarette smoking	Smoke− = non-smoking; Smoke+ − = ocasional smoking; Smoke+ + = regular smoking
Alcohol consumption	Alc = at least some alcohol consumption; NoAlc = no alcohol consumption
Beer consumption	Beer− = no beer consumption; Beer+ − = less than 1 glass daily; Beer+ = more than 1 glass daily
Wine consumption	Wine− = no wine consumption; Wine+ − = less than 1 glass daily; Wine+ = more than 1 glass daily
Consumption of spirits	Spirit− = no consumption of spirits; Spirit+ − = less than 1 glass daily; Spirit+ = more than 1 glass daily

Continued:

Variable	Coding
Health orientations	
Formal Rationality	Recoded sumscore of 2 items: FRat− = low; FRat+ − = medium; FRat+ = high formal rationality orientation
Substantive Rationality	Recoded sumscore of 3 items: SRat− SRat+ − SRat+
Health locus of control, Internal orientation	Recoded sumscore of 3 items: HlcIn− HlcIn+ − HlcIn+
Hlc Powerful others (physician orientation)	Recoded sumscore of 3 items: HlcPo− HclPo+ − HlcPo+
Hlc Chance (fatalistic orientation)	Recoded sumscore of 3 items: HlcCh− HclCh+ − HlcCh+

Note:
*Adjusted for household size

years as a standard technique for the graphical analysis of complex statistical associations. Due to its application in Bourdieu's well-known work *Distinction*, this method was first recognised by a broader audience in 1979 and started to become more popular in the 1980s. Because of its obvious advantages, this method is now also applied outside the French-speaking area. For statistically interested, yet not expert readers, correspondence analysis can be best compared to principal component or factor analysis for continuous data. As in factor analysis, a data matrix is decomposed into its eigenvalues. Simultaneously the data points are optimally projected into a low-dimensional, in most cases two-dimensional, space by a weighted least-squares criterion. (For mathematical algorithms, see Greenacre (1989) or Gifi (1990).) The aim of this kind of analysis is the visualisation of a data table that optimally reveals the relationship between the rows and columns of a two-way contingency table (Greenacre 1993). Along with the graphical display, a major advantage of this explorative technique is that it can be applied to categorical data and no assumptions of causality or general data distribution need to be made.

The basis for the following correspondence analyses are the two contingency tables with five columns (the five categories of deprivation) and thirteen rows (orientation categories) respective to seventeen rows (behaviour categories). The dimensionality of the solutions are limited by the five columns to four dimensions (Greenacre 1993). In Figures 4.5 and 4.6 the first two dimensions are plotted in a symmetrical joint plot, where column and row points are plotted in one map. Comparisons between row and column categories are possible by comparing the angles of column category and row category points with the axes or by projecting the category points on the axes and comparing their positions on a single axis. Interpreting the distance between rows and column points is not recommended, however.

Figure 4.5 shows that about 75 per cent of the data variation is covered by the first axis, 14 per cent by the second axis. The first two axes explain nearly 90 per cent of the total variation in the variable categories. Thus, the third and fourth dimensions are not relevant for interpretation. The display is stretched on a second axis. While this provides for a better visibility of the category points, the second axis appears as if it can be neglected given its rather low proportion of explained variance.

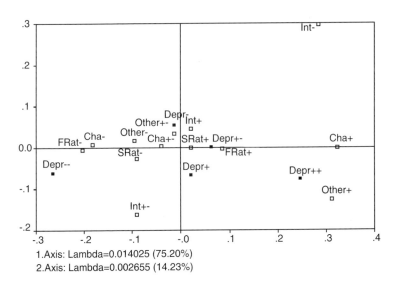

1.Axis: Lambda=0.014025 (75.20%)
2.Axis: Lambda=0.002655 (14.23%)

Figure 4.5   Correspondence analysis: deprivation and health orientations

The first dimension is strongly determined by deprivation. From low deprivation in the left to high deprivation in the right segment, the deprivation categories are spread out in an ordinal form, supporting our assumption of a hierarchical pattern in this index. It also underlines the systemic relationship between social deprivation and the health orientation variables.

With regard to the row categories the plot shows that high deprivation is related to high external (Cha+; Other+) and low internal health (Int−) locus of control. This indicates that, among the more deprived respondents orientations towards control over health are less 'internal' and more 'other' or 'chance' oriented. Respectively, the more privileged show lower scores on fatalism (Cha−). With respect to rationality orientations, the results indicate that people with higher deprivation are more likely to hold stronger normative attitudes on health behaviours. In contrast, more privileged respondents report less substantive as well as less formal rationality arguments for health behaviour regimes.

In Figure 4.6 we first observe that the ordinal distribution of our deprivation scale is again confirmed. As indicated by the Lambda coefficient, a second axis is again relatively unimportant. The pattern of the behaviour variables in the right segment of the plot indicates a rather strong relationship between high social deprivation and increased smoking and less sport activities. In the left segment of the plot, we find stronger sport participation and more wine drinkers among those in more privileged positions. Beer consumption is more equally distributed and appears less discriminating along our indicators of social conditions. The distribution of alcohol variables further suggests that in this age cohort consumption of spirits are more typical among the more privileged and that abstention is more common among respondents with higher deprivation scores. The latter results are particularly interesting indicating a differentiated pattern between alcohol consumption and relative deprivation. Of course, they require further investigation.

The purpose here was to show that one major advantage of using correspondence analysis for exploratory data analysis is that it is less restrictive with respect to our assumption about the associations between lifestyle variables, it is more open to the unexpected and can be considered more sensitive in the search for cultural variations. For example, this approach could be used to study and understand what so far have been considered 'inconsistent' health behaviour patterns. What might from a health professional perspective appear

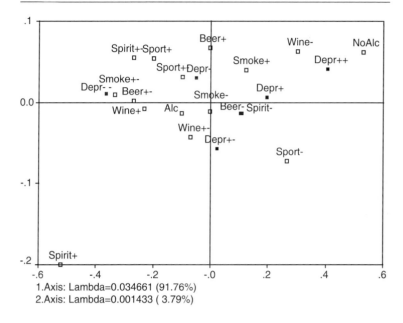

Figure 4.6   Correspondence analysis: deprivation and health
behaviour

an inconsistent pattern composed of 'no sport participation, no smoking combined with health neglecting attitudes and a rather unhealthy diet' might turn out a well-balanced health lifestyle under particular social and cultural conditions. The choices that are possible under given social and environmental circumstances might be inconsistent in a medical risk factor perspective. Yet, they could be very reasonable and health promoting under the so-called lay perspective. In that sense, we need to open our research minds and adjust our methods in order to detect more of the large variety of health relevant lifestyles.

Future directions in health lifestyle research

The line of argument and the empirical results presented in this chapter have hopefully demonstrated that sociological theory can provide helpful guidance for the development of theoretically meaningful and empirically applicable health lifestyle models. Through a sociological perspective we can conceptualise lifestyle as a social phenomenon that goes beyond relatively simple notions of risk and attach the origins of particular lifestyle behaviours to specific groups, classes and the wider society, including macro-level social processes that shape individual and collective behaviour. For instance, the finding that smoking is a major risk behaviour does not explain why certain categories of people smoke and how smoking is embedded in the social context of their lives. Studies that simply identify risk behaviours and the need to intervene to disrupt or stop these behaviours do not account for the manner in which the behaviours have become normative in a particular social context and may be related to specific social conditions. Incorporating risk behaviour patterns in a sociological perspective of lifestyles provides a more complete explanation and greater potential for understanding and addressing that behaviour.

Introducing a new concept of rationality orientations on health behaviour, the chapter should have further illustrated that traditional sociological concepts can fruitfully be applied to current health issues. The ideas and findings presented above also demonstrate, however, that we are only at the beginning of the development of more advanced models of lifestyles in the health sciences. The basic challenge for future research in that area is to comprehend theoretically and capture empirically the complex relationships between social structure and behaviour. As for empirical modelling there are a number of different approaches that can help to bridge the gap between theory and empirical measurement and testing. We have presented only one such approach that uses correspondence analysis to study the patterning of health lifestyle elements.

Many questions remain open and new questions have been raised. Specific tasks for future directions can be identified. First, the links between theory and empirical methods require improvement. We need to define theoretical criteria for the selection of appropriate health lifestyle indicators, including sociological, psychological and biological factors. Also, only on theoretical grounds can we develop convincing hypotheses about causality and reciprocity in the relationships between health lifestyle components and between lifestyles and health. Second, most studies on health and lifestyles today have been based on risk factor models. Consequently they concern only the negative aspects of health. Because health lifestyles comprise also health promoting factors, a salutogenic perspective should be developed. Third, theoretical and empirical advancements will require the development of a precisely defined and consistently applied terminology. The current practice of using

different terms differently or vaguely defined concepts synony-
mously hinders the lifestyle discourse and should be abolished.
Finally, health lifestyles are not static but complex adaptive systems.
On the individual level we can expect a certain degree of continuous
fluctuation in single lifestyle elements (e.g. people may modify their
eating patterns for rather a short term and according to particular
situations). Or, people may change their basic lifestyle pattern over
the life course, e.g. when their financial situation changes or after
experiencing major life events. On the collective level, structural
changes (e.g. employment patterns) and cultural trends promote
new health lifestyles or require giving up old ones. Therefore, we
need to develop models that help to explain stability and change in
health lifestyles.

Notes

1   The following discussion of Weber and Bourdieu had previously
appeared in Cockerham *et al.* 1997.

References

Abel T. (1991) 'Measuring health lifestyles in a comparative analysis.
Theoretical issues and empirical findings'. *Social Science and Medicine*
32: 899–908.
Abel T., Broer M., Siegrist J. (1992) 'Gesundheitsverhalten bei jungen
Erwachsenen. Empirische Analysen komplexer Verhaltensmuster und
ihrer Determinanten'. *Sozial- und Präventivmedizin* 37: 293–300.
Abel T., Cockerham W. (1993) 'Lifestyle or Lebensführung? Critical
remarks on the mistranslation of Weber's "Class, Status, Party"'. *Socio-
logical Quarterly* 34: 551–6.
Abel T., Karvonen S., Weitkunat R. (1998) 'Zur Bedeutung von Wert- und
Zweckrationalität für gesundheitsrelevanten Sport und körperliche
Aktivität. Eine explorative Analyse'. In: A. Rütten (ed.) *Public Health
und Sport*. Stuttgart: S. Nagelschmid.
Abel T., Kohlmann T. (1989) 'Health lifestyles. A comparative approach to
the culture of health concept'. In: G. Lüschen, W. Cockerham and
G. Kunz (eds) *Health and Illness in America and Germany*. München:
Oldenbourg.
Abel T., Walter E., Niemann S., Weitkunat R. (1999) 'The Bern–Munich
Lifestyle Panel. Background and baseline results from a longitudinal
health lifestyle survey'. *Sozial- und Präventivmedizin* 44: 91–106.
Bandura A. (1985) *Social Foundations of Thought and Action*. New Jersey:
Englewood Cliffs.

Berkman L. (1995) 'The role of social relations in health promotion'. *Psychosomatic Medicine* 57: 245–54.

Berkman L., Breslow L. (1983) *Health and Ways of Living: The Alameda County Study*. New York: Oxford University Press.

Blaxter M. (1990) *Health and Lifestyles*. London: Tavistock.

Bocock R. (1993) *Consumption*. London: Routledge.

Bourdieu P. (1984) *Distinction*. Cambridge: Harvard University Press.

—— (1990) *The Logic of Practice*. Stanford: Stanford University Press.

Bourdieu P., Wacquant L. (1992) *An Invitation to Reflexive Sociology*. Chicago: University of Chicago Press.

Castelli W., Anderson K. (1986) 'A population at risk. Prevalence of high cholesterol levels in hypertensive patients in the Framingham Study'. *American Journal of Medicine* 80: 23–32.

Cockerham W. (1998) 'Medical sociology'. In: N.J. Smelser (ed.) *Handbook of Sociology*. Newbury Park: Sage.

Cockerham W., Rütter A., Abel T. (1997) 'Conceptualizing contemporary health lifestyles: moving beyond Weber?'. *Sociological Quarterly* 38: 321–42.

Cockerham W., Abel T., Lüschen G. (1993) 'Max Weber, formal rationality, and health lifestyles'. *Sociological Quarterly* 34: 413–35.

Cockerham W., Lüschen G., Kunz G., Spaeth J. (1986) 'Social stratification and self-management of health'. *Journal of Health and Social Behavior* 27: 1–14.

d'Houtaud A., Field M. (1984) 'The image of health. Variations in perception by social class in a French population'. *Sociology of Health and Illness* 6: 30–59.

Dahrendorf R. (1979) *Life Chances*. Chicago: University of Chicago Press.

Dean K. (1993) 'Integrating theory and methods in population health research'. In: K. Dean (ed.) *Population Health Research*. London: Sage.

Featherstone M. (1991) *Consumer Culture and Postmodernism*. London: Sage.

Giddens A. (1991) *Modernity and Self-identity*. Stanford: Stanford University Press.

Gifi A. (1990) *Nonlinear Multivariate Analysis*. Chichester: Wiley.

Greenacre M. (1989) *Theory and Applications of Correspondence Analysis*. New York: Academic Press.

—— (1993) *Correspondence Analysis in Practice*. London: Academic Press.

Harris D., Guten S. (1979) 'Health-protective behavior. An exploratory study'. *Journal of Health and Social Behavior* 20: 17–29.

Haug M. and Lavin B. (1981) 'Practitioner or patient – who's in charge?' *Journal of Health and Social Behavior* 22: 212–29.

Hayes D., Ross C. (1987) 'Concern with appearance, health beliefs, and eating habits'. *Journal of Health and Social Behavior* 28: 17–29.

Jenkins R. (1992) *Pierre Bourdieu*. London: Routledge.

Kickbusch I. (1986) 'Life-styles and health'. *Social Science and Medicine* 22: 117–23.

Kooiker S., Christiansen T. (1995) 'Inequalities in health. The interaction of circumstances and health related behaviour'. *Sociology of Health and Illness* 17: 495–524.

Macintyre S. (1997) 'The Black Report and beyond. What are the issues?' *Social Science and Medicine* 44: 723–45.

McQueen D. (1987) 'A research program in lifestyle and health. Methodological and theoretical considerations'. *Revue d'Epidemiologie et de Santé Publique* 35: 28–35.

Mechanic D., Cleary P. (1980) 'Factors associated with the maintenance of positive health behavior'. *Preventive Medicine* 9: 805–14.

Noack H. (1988) 'Measuring health behaviour and health. Towards new health promotion indicators'. *Health Promotion* 3: 5–11.

Puska P., Tuomilehto J., Nissinen A., Vartiainen E. (eds) (1995) *The North Karelia Project. 20 years Results and Experiences.* Helsinki: National Public Health Institute.

Siegrist J. (1995) *Medizinische Soziologie*, 5th edition. Munich: Urban und Schwarzenberg.

Townsend P. (1979) *Poverty in the United Kingdom. A Survey of Household Resources and Standards of Living.* Harmondsworth: Penguin Books.

Uitenbroek D. (1993) 'Relationships between leisure time physical activity for exercise and other health related behaviours'. *Sozial- und Präventivmedizin* 38: 356–61.

Weber M. (1946) *From Max Weber. Essays in Sociology.* New York: Oxford University Press.

—— (1978) *Economy and Society.* Berkeley: University of California Press.

WHO MONICA Project Principal Investigators (1988) 'The World Health Organization MONICA Project (monitoring trends and determinants in cardiovascular disease). A major international collaboration'. *Journal of Clinical Epidemiology* 41: 105–14.

Wrong D. (1990) The influence of sociological ideas on American culture. In: H.J. Gans (ed.) *Sociology in America.* Newbury Park, CA: Sage.

Part II

Methodological challenges

Forming a bridge between the agenda-setting emphasis of Part I and the methodological concerns of Part II, Chapter 5 by Dale Webb and David Wright explores the implications of the postmodernist perspective for evaluating effectiveness in health promotion. Drawing on findings from focus group interviews with health promotion providers and purchasers, the authors propose that there is an affinity between postmodernism and health promotion, as evidenced by a common concern with embracing positive health (rather than disease), questioning the discourse of causality, celebrating multiple perspectives and subjectivity, championing multi-disciplinarity, and valuing diversity and fragmentation over universality and generalisability. The chapter considers what constitutes a postmodern approach to health promotion research and practice, focusing on: research methods, the notion of causality, indicators of success, and the language of health care evaluation. It is argued that, while a postmodern mode of enquiry can serve as a useful corrective of the positivist, outcome-driven biomedical model, there are some limitations to this approach. The chapter concludes with a call to develop a pluralistic framework for health promotion research which attempts to transcend the current positivist *versus* post-positivist paradigm wars.

Chapter 6 by Paul Flowers, Jamie Frankis and Graham Hart takes up the challenge laid down by Webb and Wright by adopting 'a multi-method approach ... encompassing different epistemological frameworks (positivism and phenomenology)' in order to evaluate a peer-led, community-level intervention (the Gay Men's Task Force initiative) to promote sexual health among gay men in Glasgow. It outlines the evaluative technologies employed within four key stages in evaluation: development work; formative evaluation; process evaluation; and outcome evaluation. The authors describe the various methods they adopted to address the specific questions raised at each stage in the evaluation process, including participant observation, self-administered questionnaires, individual in-depth interviews, focus group discussions and self-complete diaries. The differing kinds of evidence produced by these disparate approaches are discussed in terms of the notion of intervention utility (efficacy, transferability and sustainability).

In Chapter 7 Elisabeth Fosse reports the findings of research into the implementation of a national programme in Norway, which was intended to enhance intersectoral co-operation and stimulate municipalities to give higher priority to health promotion. The theoretical framework adopted by the author seeks to combine a decision-making (top down) perspective and a process (bottom up) perspective, with a view to illuminating the roles of both actors and organisations in implementing the programme. Data were gathered using qualitative methods at municipal, regional and national levels. There was only one municipality in which the project continued to receive funding after the programme period was over, while in three municipalities there was no organisational change at all. Implementation theory highlights some of the reasons why the programme had such limited impacts. Taking a decision-making perspective, factors of internal organisation seemed to be especially important in explaining the lack of implementation. In a process perspective, the role of health professionals at local and national levels appeared to be important. Intersectoral co-operation was most successful when the health professionals acted as 'co-players'. Where they chose the role of controllers, co-operation did not work so well. The author concludes that the health services should not play a dominant part in health promotion policy. To secure a more holistic approach, health promotion should be organised as an intersectoral field.

In Chapter 8 Janine Hale explores the relationship between health economics and health promotion. Policy planners in the health care sector recognise the inevitability of having to make difficult choices, as a result of the scarcity of resources, and increasingly rely on the principle of efficiency when so doing. Demonstrating that an intervention is effective is no longer sufficient; it is vital to assess the cost of achieving an effect. The (main) objective of health care, however, is to produce health and health can be produced in many ways other than through the formal health care sector, for example through health promotion. It is often stated that when health economists apply the standard economic appraisal techniques to health promotion, they are discriminating against it or selling it short. The chapter outlines the role health economics can play in helping to evaluate health promotion programmes and to illustrate the difficulties encountered when applying the standard economic evaluation techniques, such as discounting, length of follow-up, identification and measurement of benefits. The chapter argues that any difficulties can only be overcome through collaboration between economists and health promotion specialists/researchers. The chapter also illuminates the role of health economics in understanding individual decision-making relating to health relevant behaviour.

Chapter 5

Postmodernism and health promotion

Implications for the debate on effectiveness

Dale Webb and David Wright

Introduction

This chapter considers the value of a postmodern perspective to understanding health promotion and the current debate on measuring its effectiveness. Although health promotion has developed from a mix of positivist disciplines – for example, medicine, epidemiology and behavioural psychology – and constructivist disciplines such as community development and community psychology (Labonte and Robertson 1996), it may be that the dominant tenets of health promotion are more consistent with the constructivist underpinnings of postmodernism than the positivist premises of evidence-based health care. If so, a postmodernist mode of enquiry can serve as a useful corrective to the outcomes research model in measuring the effectiveness of health promotion.

This chapter starts from an observation that the debate in professional health promotion journals on measuring effectiveness has largely been argued at the level of research methodology, and has crystallised around what at times have been fairly polarised views on the use of randomised controlled trials (RCTs) in health promotion research. With some notable exceptions (for example, Poland 1992, Kelly and Charlton 1995), what those debates have not done is to examine the philosophical assumptions that underpin methodological choices. This is crucial because important methodological problems cannot be resolved unless those concerned with health promotion research engage with its underlying epistemology. What postmodernism can offer health promotion is a lens through which it is possible to view these epistemological questions and relate them to its research and practice. It also serves as a useful corrective of the biomedical model in health promotion. Whilst it may be true that evaluation, as a research discipline, needs 'another round of positivism bashing like a hole in the head' (Pawson and Tilley 1997: xiv–xv), this is arguably not the case in health promotion, given that the debate has been less well developed than in other fields.

Health promotion as a postmodern endeavour?

The term 'postmodernism' is frequently used to describe events and expressions of contemporary social culture. Fifteen years on from Lyotard's (1984) famous treatise on the subject, everything seems to be postmodern. Architecture (e.g. Phillip Johnson and Terry Farrell), art (e.g. Rauschenberg and Salle), music (e.g. Schnittke and Berio) and even Vic Reeves and Bob Mortimer's BBC2 panel-game spoof, *Shooting Stars*, are given the epithet of being postmodern. So popular has this term become that postmodernism appears to be the automatic theoretical justification for all that is confused, unconventional and bizarre. Within this climate, it is not surprising that health promotion, itself a complex concern, has begun to consider issues of postmodernism (Peterson and Bunton 1997, Fox 1991).

Rather than simply applying and accepting postmodern concepts to health promotion, this section seeks to illuminate exactly what is meant by postmodernism, how this relates to developments in health promotion, and the extent to which earlier frameworks in health promotion were modern endeavours. In order to achieve this, it is necessary not only to explore the conceptual frameworks underpinning postmodernism and its modernist counterpart, but also to engage with the historical context of these approaches.

Modernism, positivism and methods in health research

The impact of modernism on Western society has been marked in many areas of cultural experience. Modernist enterprises are clearly distinguished in areas of art (Picasso, Braque), architecture (Le Corbusier, Mies van der Rohe), music (Stravinsky, Schoenberg) and literature (Joyce, Eliot), but it is a little confusing to consider precisely why health related research should be associated with these cultural trends.

Modernism was born out of Cartesian, Enlightenment philosophies: a belief in the functioning of a rational, objective and scientific mind as an interpretative tool in understanding the external world. Early modern, scientific thought can be found in the writings of Francis Bacon (1561–1626), a philosopher credited as being the founder of 'inductivism'. Inductivists believed that universal statements, such as hypotheses, can be derived from singular statements, such as experimentation. Reacting against these inductivist assertions, Descartes and Leibniz developed a 'deductivist' framework in which singular statements are derived from universal considerations.

Fundamentally, the belief in the scientific approach centred on the assertion that facts exist independently of the observer and that they can be identified through experience and observation. Descartes commented on this experiential basis to scientific enquiry in his famous treatise *Discourse on Method* (1637):

> while I decided thus to think that everything was false, it followed necessarily that I who thought must be something; and observing that this truth: I think, therefore I am, was so certain and so evident that all the most extravagant suppositions of the sceptics were not capable of shaking it, I judged that I could accept it without scruple as the first principle of the philosophy I was seeking.
>
> (Descartes, 1968: 53–4)

Positivism, developed during the nineteenth century in the writings of August Comte (1798–1857), furthered these ideas, perceiving human social phenomena to be structured in the same way as the natural inorganic and organic world. Hence social considerations could also be explored scientifically.

The foundation of modernism is closely related to these scientific and positivist concerns, perceiving the (social and physical) world to be structured in a complex and confusing array of processes which required a unitary and detached examination to craft order in a disorderly world. Or as Habermas puts it, modernity aims 'to develop objective science, universal morality and law, and autonomous art according to their inner logic' (Habermas 1983: 9).

Consequently, modernism reveres methodology as a means to create security against epistemological insecurity. That is to say, experimental design and observation can be used to understand a complex social reality.

Health can similarly be seen to be a complex social phenomenon requiring a coherent, experimental methodological design to contend with the varied possibilities of health attainment. This requirement has become an imperative in contemporary research with the Cochrane Collaboration's (1994) recommended use of experimental studies employing control or comparison groups. These 'randomised controlled trials' were thought to minimise bias and thus generate more meaningful and reliable evidence for the effectiveness of health care interventions. Randomised controlled trials were heralded as a 'gold standard', given their ability to ensure that experimental and control groups are socially equivalent, that unknown factors influencing outcomes are equally distributed between groups, and that the possibility of researcher bias is minimised (Oakley *et al.* 1996, Lawrence *et al.* 1989).

Given this concern of using scientifically validated, positivist RCT methodological techniques to minimise the limitations derived from epistemological complexities, the dominant model of health care evaluation can be considered to be a modernistic endeavour.

Postmodernism and the critique of positivist methodologies of health research

The growth of modernist ideals from the sixteenth century to the beginning of this century was associated with significant social optimism. The development of science and the principles of the Enlightenment were believed to provide great benefits to society. The onset of the Industrial Revolution and advancement of medicine were just two ways in which science and modernity were seen to be a cure-all for social ills. This confidence was reflected well in the Great Exhibition in 1851, where the latest technological developments were presented as a mark of confidence and pride for the future.

However, this optimism quickly eroded throughout the twentieth century. The rise to power of Adolf Hitler, the Second World War and the aftermath of the Hiroshima and Nagasaki bombings all demonstrated the destructive potential of technological development. Earlier, the destruction of densely populated areas of Paris by Haussman in the mid-nineteenth century through the construction of the *grands boulevards* was seen to be a sanitisation of social complexity through technology (Harvey 1985). Similarly, the redevelopment of the Bronx in New York by Robert Moses was perceived to reflect the demolition of social life through corporate development (Berman 1983). In London during the 1960s, the collapse of Ronan's Point severely questioned the government's housing policy and the safety of modern urban development in rectifying housing problems (Hutchinson 1988). Against these historical events, there developed 'a rage against humanism and the Enlightenment legacy' (Bernstein 1985: 25).

Several cultural critics have suggested that these failures derive from the separation of modernity from modernism (Habermas 1983, Berman 1983, Harvey 1989). This is to say, the ideology of modernity is believed to be sound and supportive of social needs, whereas the practice (as reflected in Haussman, Moses and the 1960s UK housing policy) is seen to be destructive of those goals. Others, however, consider modernity to be irrevocably flawed in its bypassing of chaotic social reality through the (false) belief in methodological security (Lyotard 1984). In other words, if social reality is marked by complexity, flux and change, as postmodernists argue, then any methodological desire for order and singularity is delusional. Thus, the postmodern movement became established to reject the methodological enlightenment of a complex epistemology, and to celebrate and rejoice in the diversity, fragmentation and chaos of the social world.

In this regard, Jencks (1984) dates the birth of postmodern architecture to 3:32 p.m. on 15 July 1972, when the modernist Pruitt-Igoe housing development in St Louis was destroyed on the basis of being an uninhabitable dwelling for the people it housed. The singular, 'meta' narrative expression of architectural design was seen to be incompatible with social living. In place of the modern paradigm, postmodernism embraced the 'multi' narratives of social existence. In architecture, this meant utilising pastiche, reproduction, fragmentation, humour, juxtaposition and chaos to reflect disordered social processes. Thus Quinlan Terry's Richmond Riverside Panorama constructed in the 1980s revives past urban forms with the imitation of eighteenth-century classicism (Hutchinson 1988). Alternatively, Charles Moore's *Piazza d'Italia* in New Orleans uses pastiche, humour and façadism to create his archetypally postmodern piece of architecture.

The growth in technological advancement, particularly in the areas of finance and telecommunication, furthered this sense of disorientation, with the experiential reduction of spatial difference, what Harvey (1989) has referred to as the effects of 'time–space compression'. Associated with these trends were rising inflation in world markets, the raising of oil prices by OPEC and the Arab decision to embargo oil exports to the West in 1973. This had the effect of driving technological and organisational change, and for increasing the impetus for business to seek employees on the global stage (Harvey 1989).

Intriguingly, the growth of health promotion during the 1970s and the critique of the earlier biomedical framework of opposing health against disease situates well with these broader cultural trends (Antonovsky 1996, Macdonald and Bunton 1992). In particular, the Lalonde report of 1974 and the 1978 Alma Ata declaration on primary health care were significant in critiquing the view of health as a discrete quantifiable variable, advocating instead consideration of the social and cultural context of health (Lalonde 1974, WHO 1978, Tones and Tilford 1994).

In 1984, the World Health Organization established a programme of health promotion and published a discussion document on the concept and principles of health promotion (WHO 1984) which became crystallised in the Ottawa Charter of 1986 (WHO 1986). The Charter declared that:

> Health promotion is the process of enabling people to increase control over, and improve, their health ... to identify and to realise aspirations, to satisfy needs, and to change or cope with the environment. Health is seen, therefore, as a resource for everyday life, not the objective of living. Health is a positive concept emphasising social and personal resources, as well as physical capabilities.
>
> (WHO 1986)

It is this appeal to concepts of health as a 'resource for everyday life' which reflects postmodern sentiments. No longer should health just be seen to be a complex social reality, but methodological enquiries should seek to reflect rather than order these concerns. More recently, the Jakarta Declaration on Health Promotion into the twenty-first century has emphasised the need to promote social responsibility for health, for a consolidation and expansion of partnerships for health, and for increased community capacity to influence the determinants of health.

These trends in health promotion reflect a shift away from singular, quantifiable and positivist definitions of health as the opposite of disease to an engagement with the social complexity and contingency of health care considerations. Given this desire to relate health concerns to the diversity and convoluted nature of everyday life, rather than appealing defensively to the sanctity of a single scientific method, health research can be seen to be a profoundly postmodern endeavour.

Defining health and the limits of postmodernism

Within a postmodern mode of enquiry, health is seen to be a multiply determined, culturally contingent concern. Research on health promotion, therefore, has to perceive health not as an unwavering scientific fact or universal truth, but rather as a concept constructed within and dependent upon a chaotic and diverse social reality. However, as several notable commentators on social theory have shown (Jameson 1984, Huyssens 1984, Harvey 1989, 1996, Bauman 1997), there exist certain fatal flaws within postmodernism.

First, in rejecting the use of coherent methodologies to decipher complex epistemologies, postmodernists have gone too far in the opposite direction, prioritising chaotic social process above the need to articulate coherent and workable frameworks of analysis. Consequently, postmodernism denies the very methodological tools needed to be able to consider the applicability or the relevance of postmodern modes of thought (Featherstone 1989). Hence, postmodernism can only justify itself in a tautologous fashion: the world is postmodern because it is postmodern. In this regard, postmodernism is self-contradictory. In order to speak or write postmodern, one has to adopt a voice from somewhere and speak within a narrative order that contradicts postmodernism's rejection of singular ('meta') narratives. Harvey (1989) similarly states that there is nothing more totalising than a framework that rejects all other modes of analysis on the basis of perceiving them to be totalising.

Second, postmodernism can be an intensely disempowering and apolitical enterprise. Adopting a relativistic, 'anything goes' standpoint means that there can be no basis from which to assess the validity or relevance of one voice above another. Fascistic discourse must therefore be given equal weight to feminist perspectives. To mediate or judge one in relation to the other would be to impose a hierarchy that contradicts the postmodern framework. Similarly, there is something politically suspicious about a line of enquiry in which marginalised voices within research find themselves silenced by a sentiment which perceives any voice to be contrary to the ideals of postmodern 'multi-vocality' (Miller 1986, McDowell 1992). As Haraway argues: 'Some differences are playful; some are poles of world historical systems of domination. Epistemology is about knowing the difference' (Haraway 1991: 560).

This relativistic standpoint of 'anything goes', whereby all information generated would be equally valid, has been criticised by some health promotion researchers as a means of producing a confused and impossibly dense set of research data. Stevenson and Burke (1992), for example, suggest that such an approach would dilute what they see as an already desultory research practice. Meaning becomes 'relegated' to

> the different needs, values and interpretations of endlessly differentiated communities, so that health promotion indicators of healthy communities provide only an 'indication but not an explanation of the state of a particular community'.
> (Stevenson and Burke 1992: S51, citing Hayes and Willms 1990)

A further aspect of this depoliticised consequence of postmodernism was described by Harvey (1996) in his account of a fire at the Imperial Foods chicken-processing plant in Hamlet, North Carolina (1996). Twenty-five workers died in the fire due to insufficient safety procedures and the locking of the emergency exit. However, given that most of the workers were either underpaid, female or black, the reaction to the fire resulted in fragmentary political groups forming around issues of class, race and gender. None of these groups worked together, and thus a coherent, politically powerful force was lost to the tensions and confusions of the 'multiple voices'. This, Harvey felt, was a perfect reflection of the need to adopt a coherent standpoint at a time of social need, and thus of the need to reject postmodern ideals in favour of modernist principles.

Third, related to this, at a methodological level, postmodernism rejects the possibility of constructing strategically coherent areas of research. For example, in his critique of epidemiological studies of HIV and AIDS, Brown (1995) suggests that quantitative, positivist approaches are useful in providing accessible and visually meaningful forms of representation. Likewise, Young (1990, 1995) argues that a concern for postmodern diversity should not render the aims of social justice and equality redundant. In relation to health care concerns, the call for diversity and plurality within concepts of health promotion and education should not undermine the strategic importance of coherent forms of medical research and health care evaluation.

Therefore, whilst postmodernism is useful in serving as a critique for the automatic assumption that there are correct ways of 'doing research', nevertheless the limitations of postmodern lines of enquiry need to be considered. What is important, therefore, is to appreciate that no approach to health promotion is inherently right or wrong, and that it is the context in which health related research, whether it is in the form of RCTs or more qualitative methodologies, are conducted that has to be made evident. It is this strategic, contextual approach to health promotion that needs to be developed.

The implications of the postmodern critique for health promotion

What is the key postmodern health promotion concept?

Now that the philosophical underpinnings of postmodernism and modernism have been outlined, it is necessary to consider in more detail how these issues are played out in specific relation to health promotion. Postmodernists would suggest that the conceptual key for health promotion is positive health, emphasising an individual's personal and social, as well as physical, capacities (Kelly *et al.* 1993). In a postmodern approach, health is viewed not as the opposite of disease, which is a dichotomy characteristic of modernist social theory, but as something which changes and adapts to one's environment. Health is a resource for everyday life, which represents a significant departure from a conception of health as an absence of disease. The challenge is for health promotion to articulate clearly that reductivist methodologies are inappropriate for measuring positive health and for it to develop end-points consistent with this new approach. However, postmodernists also caution that the concept of positive health should not be articulated within the kind of systemic view that characterises a modernist approach to social life. A systemic view of positive health understands it to be a function of macro-level systems rather than micro-level ones (Kelly and Charlton 1995). Postmodernists argue that the social world is too chaotic to be understood that way, and maintain that conceptual-ising positive health as a function of systems blinds health promotion researchers and practitioners to aspects of health that may lie outside of those systems. Thus, the postmodern critique calls for a willingness to anticipate the unexpected, and to frame health promotion research methodologies according to the intervention and not the intervention according to the research methodology.

Causality versus intertextuality – rationality and irrationality

Logical positivism subscribes to the notion of a single reality which is independent of any observer, a reality which is driven by universal, discoverable laws and truths that exist independent of time and space. These truths can be understood at least in principle, through a mechanical explanation of cause and effect (Guba 1990). Recently, critical realists have attempted to move the debate forward (Pawson and Tilley 1997) in their attention to understanding the contexts in which interventions take place. Pawson and Tilley (1997), citing Sayer (1994), argue that 'the relationship between causal mecha-nisms and their effects is not fixed, but contingent' (69).

Their concern with the '*contextual conditioning* of causal mecha-nisms' (69, original emphasis) holds little sway with postmodernists who eschew a realist ontology: in the arena of health policy inter-ventions, the idea that a context can be anything other than constantly fluid is rejected.

Many postmodernists take up positions which oppose the notion of a single truth and which are anti-causal. They argue that the search for 'evidence' is illusory because, even if a single reality does exist, our understanding of it can only ever be a social construct. Postmodernism's principal strategy is deconstruction (Derrida 1978), an approach which dismisses singular considerations of social processes (or texts) in favour of engaging with the diverse readings and experiences of those processes (or texts). Furthermore, a deconstructive approach enables the researcher to embrace the contradictions inherent within social processes, illustrating how social (con)texts are interdependent with other (con)texts, that is to say, they are intertextual.

However, there is a need for further theorisation in this area. Confusion about how, and in what contexts, health promotion can be understood through causal perspectives was noted in a recent study of the perceptions of health promotion practitioners and commissioners about current approaches to determining effectiveness in health promotion (Webb 1997). Study participants asserted that health promotion could not *easily* relate to a causal view of the social world, but also suggested that the function of intermediate outcome measures is that they can represent a path in a causal chain. For example, a ban on the advertising of tobacco products is an important intermediate measure for a reduction in coronary heart disease as it is known to lead to a reduction of consumption levels, which is widely believed to lead to reductions in premature mortality and morbidity. However, there was no discussion about whether health promotion should *reject* causal perspectives, and if so, what this might mean for understanding health promotion activities.

What constitutes admissible data? – objectivity and subjectivity

The critique of the metanarrative is an important one – the idea that scientific paradigms are constructed to define complete or 'totalising' social processes and phenomena: 'Each of these metanarratives contends it is validated on the basis of external criteria, while all of them, postmodernists suggest, are really dependent on a system of internal self-validating logic' (Rosenau 1994: 305).

Thus, the idea that all research should be objective is not an external truth written in stone but a construct of the positivist paradigm. Medical science is one such metanarrative. Labonte and Robertson (1996) argue that social relations of power, in which certain kinds of knowledge are legitimised and others are not, are embedded in these metanarratives. Thus, work which is part of standard, scientific enquiry is funded and disseminated more easily than that taking unconventional approaches (Lincoln 1992). Moreover, the objectivity of the biomedical model has been criticised for treating the social world in such a way as to rob it of its historical and intersubjective roots (Poland 1992). In contrast, a postmodernist framework embraces multiple narratives, reflecting a range of perspectives and interests. It seeks to characterise particular narratives as 'discourses' that reveal the speakers' cultural values and place in the dominant power structure (Fox 1991). Effectiveness would then be measured, not according to a comparison group-based experimental model, but by those engaged in the process of designing and using their own programmes for health gain, as they have defined it.

Order and disorder – discipline imperialism and interdisciplinarity

Positivist research is characterised by a discipline-led model and is based on foundationalism – the notion that knowledge is founded in disciplines – which attempts to simplify the social world by asserting artificial disciplinary boundaries within which research is conducted (Usher 1996). This can be understood as an attempt to bring order to a disorderly world (Tones and Tilford 1994). Postmodernism challenges foundationalism and posits that knowledge formation is interdisciplinary. This is another way in which health promotion is more consistent with postmodernism than positivism. One has only to think of the importance attached in health promotion to working in health alliances, to Healthy Cities initiatives and to the WHO Health for All initiative to realise that health promotion is a multi-disciplinary endeavour. The interdisciplinary nature of health promotion is well understood in the field, in which specialist health promotion is viewed as one component of a multi- or transdisciplinary endeavour. Thus, the challenge is to develop a consensus on the ownership of measures, that is, on an understanding of whose performance should be evaluated. However, it is also the case that some in health promotion, echoing modernist ideas, also want to see specialist health promotion emerging as a distinct discipline, lending it strength and credibility, particularly in the eyes of their biomedical colleagues.

A search for indicators – universality and generalisability

Positivism understands research as a universal process in which a set of general methods is applied. The test of knowledge in positivism is its generalisability and predictive power, whereas postmodern approaches lend primacy to interpretive power, meaning and illumination (Usher 1996). The postmodern method favours a comprehensive characterisation of multiple perspectives over a reductive approach to intervention and evaluation. Postmodernist methodologies seek to permit diverse opinion and fragmentary processes, perceiving this disorder to relate more to the reality of responding to diverse health promotion needs instead of focusing on a single goal or desirable outcome. Postmodern philosophy rejects operationalising complex concepts such as empowerment or well-being as *simple indicators*, given that a postmodern view posits that there is no absolute truth about health and that positive health is a quality defined by individuals and groups, not imposed by external forces.

A postmodern approach to health promotion research and practice

What, then, would health promotion practice and research look like, if the postmodern premises were accepted more explicitly by commissioners and providers? With regard to practice, health promotion is already committed to the idea that health is a multiply determined, multi-dimensional concept (Rubenstein *et al.* 1989), and that the role of health promotion is to help meet some of the diverse needs and aspirations of different communities. If health is a resource for living, then it is difficult to see how a unifying definition of this can be derived. A postmodern approach to health promotion research would concern itself with four key issues: research methods; the notion of causality; the search for indicators of success; and the language of health care evaluation.

Research methods

Development is required with regard to hierarchies of evidence. Rather than automatically setting RCTs at the top and qualitative studies at the bottom, health promotion research values would be better driven by the questions being asked. For simple interventions in relatively closed systems for which valid short-term outcomes exist, RCTs may provide the most appropriate evaluative tool. However, qualitative methods will be preferred when the goal is to explicate and illuminate process. It is understandable that some commentators (Macdonald 1996) have called for a research hierarchy of *qualitative methods* which might be seen to lend credibility in the minds of those working to the Cochrane hierarchy. However, such a notion would be rejected by many postmodernists – given a commitment to different truths, there can be no single method which is universally 'best' for discovering those truths (Webb 1999). What is important is to develop standards for the design, implementation and reporting of qualitative studies in health promotion.

Indeed, work has been underway with a small multi-disciplinary team of social science researchers at the Health Education Authority who have been attempting to develop a consensus on what constitutes a rigorous approach to qualitative research (Meyrick and Gillies 1998), and a health technology review has now been published that synthesises different schools of thought in this regard (Murphy *et al.* 1998).

Causality

The issue of causality is important to the future direction of health promotion research. Health promotion may be reaching an epistemological turning point, where it is beginning to uproot itself from positivism. However, it is also possible that health promotion is beginning to understand how its epistemological contradictions can be accommodated in a new way. Health promotion does not need to reject the notion of causality outright. Given the diversity of health promotion interventions it seems reasonable to subscribe to the view that in some areas it is possible to understand what takes place in a causal way. But it is also possible to think of the intertextuality of health promotion and the interdependence of a number of social processes through which health is affected. This influences whether research methods should be employed which can best determine causal relationships or those which can best illuminate social processes.

Indicators of success

A postmodern approach to health promotion research suggests that the search for universal indicators of success is premised on an epistemology which fails to situate social life:

> If one concedes that circumstances giving rise to conditions in one community are not the same as those operating in another, then the validity of employing indicators that would allow for comparison with other communities may be questioned on the grounds that neither the baselines, nor the processes, are truly comparable.
>
> (Hayes and Willms 1990: 165)

The evaluation of many key health promotion concepts is problematic unless, as Kelly *et al.* (1993) suggest, it is understood that those concepts are best defined subjectively. Thus, the application of positivist, rationalist methods (i.e., standardised measures) would not be accepted as appropriate.

The language of health care evaluation

Finally, it has been argued that the dominant framework in health care evaluation is health economics. Burrows *et al.* (1995) refer to health economics as a modernist discourse that is being applied to the evaluation of a postmodern project (that is, health promotion). In a subsequent article Burrows (1996) went on to clarify that the discourse of health economics has provided a vocabulary to the internal market of the NHS which is characterised by aims, inputs and measurable objectives. He argued that health promotion providers have had difficulties articulating and evaluating their practice within such a template, but that they have had to appropriate this discourse in order to compete for scarce resources. The danger is, he said, that 'in so doing it is likely that the nature of health promotion practice will be transformed as those interventions better able to conform to dominant contractual templates will be given priority' (366).

In Webb's (1997) study, participants expressed frustration in having to articulate their practice in this way, suggesting that, although it might lend them greater credibility and possibly gain extra funding, it is actually of limited practical use. Further, postmodernism critiques the epistemology of a discourse on evidence based health, which has positivist tendencies, and promotes a discourse on knowledge based health, which suggests a plurality of rationalities, characteristic of a postmodern approach to understanding social life.

Conclusion

It has been argued that there are natural affinities between postmodernism and health promotion, and that what postmodernism can offer health promotion is a lens through which to critique the philosophical assumptions that underpin research paradigms. It provokes consideration about the relationship between a biomedical model of health and a socio-environmental one. It encourages health promotion researchers and practitioners to re-frame arguments about the role of different research methods, and it casts doubt on the enterprise for evidence as expressed as a singular rationality. Although it does not intend to improve upon that which it deconstructs, it does offer significant insights for health promotion. But ultimately, it refuses to move on from deconstruction to reconstructing a research framework, and therefore it is difficult to reconcile postmodern ideals with the need to articulate and express a consistent research method. Although the epistemologies of positivism and constructivism seem antithetical in principle, the mixed heritage of health promotion lends itself to an evaluative strategy that can build on both process and outcome based methods, depending on the question asked. The contested nature of health promotion's epistemology may be a consequence of the newness of its emerging discipline status, where epistemological struggles are inevitable. In this context, parallels with other new disciplines such as nursing may be drawn (Usher 1996). The challenge, therefore, is to develop a pluralistic framework for health promotion research that acknowledges the importance of accommodating difference about the basic premises of health care evaluation, and that can develop an understanding of the relationship between conflicting paradigms which attempts to resolve tension and identify common themes and purposes.

References

Antonovsky A. (1996) 'The salutogenic model as a theory to guide health promotion'. *Health Promotion International* 11: 11–18

Bauman Z. (1997) *Postmodernity and its Discontents*. Cambridge: Polity.

Berman M. (1983) *All That's Solid Melts into Air*. London: Verso.

Bernstein R. (ed.) (1985) *Habermas and Modernity*. Oxford: Polity Press.

Brown M. (1995) 'Ironies of distance: an ongoing critique of the geographies of AIDS'. *Environment and Planning D: Society and Space* 13: 159–83.

Burrows R. (1996) 'Health promotion and the vocabulary of the internal market'. *Health Education Research* 11: 365–6.

Burrows R., Bunton R., Muncer S., Gillen K. (1995) 'The efficacy of health promotion, health economics and late modernism'. *Health Education Research* 10: 241–9.

Cochrane Collaboration (1994) *Report*. Oxford: Cochrane Centre.

Derrida J. (1978) *Writing and Difference*. London: Routledge and Kegan Paul.

Descartes R. (1968) *Discourse on Method, and the Meditations.* Harmondsworth: Penguin.

Featherstone M. (1989) 'Towards a sociology of postmodern culture'. In: H. Haferkamp (ed.) *Social Structure and Culture.* Amsterdam: de Gruyter Press.

Fox N. (1991) 'Postmodernism, rationality and the evaluation of health care'. *Sociological Review* 39: 709–44.

Guba E. (1990) 'The alternative paradigm dialog'. In: E. Guba (ed.) *The Paradigm Dialog.* California: Sage.

Habermas J. (1983) 'Modernity: an incomplete project'. In: H. Foster (ed.) *The Anti-Aesthetic: Essays on Postmodern Culture.* Washington: Port Townsend.

Haraway D. (1991) *Simians, Cyborgs and Women: The Reinvention of Nature.* London: Free Association Books.

Harvey D. (1985) *Consciousness and the Urban Experience: Studies in the History and Theory of Capitalist Urbanization.* Oxford: Blackwell.

—— (1989) *The Condition of Postmodernity: An Enquiry into the Origins of Cultural Change.* Oxford: Blackwell.

—— (1996) *Justice, Nature and the Geography of Difference.* Oxford: Blackwell.

Hayes M., Willms S. (1990) 'Healthy community indicators: the perils of the search and the paucity of the find'. *Health Promotion International* 5: 161–6.

Hutchinson M. (1988) *The Prince of Wales – Right or Wrong?* London: Faber and Faber.

Huyssens A. (1984) 'Mapping the post-modern'. *New German Critique* 33: 5–52.

Jameson F. (1984) 'Postmodernism, or the cultural logic of late capitalism'. *New Left Review* 146: 53–92.

Jencks C. (1984) *The Language of Post-Modern Architecture.* London: Academy Editions.

Kelly P., Charlton B. (1995) 'The modern and the postmodern in health promotion'. In: R. Bunton, S. Nettleton, R. Burrows (eds) *The Sociology of Health Promotion: Critical Analyses of Consumption, Lifestyle and Risk.* Routledge: London.

Kelly P., Davies J., Charlton B. (1993) 'Healthy cities: a modern problem or a post-modern solution?' In: J. Davies and M. Kelly (eds) *Healthy Cities: Research and Practice.* Routledge: London.

Labonte R., Robertson A. (1996) 'Delivering the goods, showing our stuff: the case for a constructivist paradigm for health promotion research and practice'. *Health Education Quarterly* 23: 431–47.

Lalonde M. (1974) *A New Perspective on the Health of Canadians. A Working Document.* Canada.

Lawrence R., Friedman G., DeFriese G. *et al.* (1989) *Guide to Clinical Preventive Services: An Assessment of the Effectiveness of 169*

Interventions – Report of the U.S. Preventive Services Task Force. Maryland: Williams and Wilkins.

Lincoln Y. (1992) 'Fourth generation evaluation, the paradigm revolution and health promotion'. *Canadian Journal of Public Health* 83 (Supplement 1): S6–S10.

Lyotard J. (1984) *The Postmodern Condition*. Manchester: Manchester University Press.

Macdonald G. (1996) 'Where next for evaluation?' *Health Promotion International* 11: 171–3.

Macdonald G., Bunton R. (1992) 'Health promotion: discipline or disciplines?' In: R. Bunton and G. Macdonald (eds) *Health Promotion: Disciplines and Diversity*. London: Routledge.

McDowell L. (1992) 'Multiple voices: speaking from inside and outside "the project"'. *Antipode* 24: 56–72.

Meyrick J., Gillies P. (1998) 'Recognising the contribution of qualitative studies to systematic reviews and the search for evidence in health promotion: not widening the goal posts but changing the field of play' (unpublished consultation paper). London: Health Education Authority.

Miller N. (1986) 'Changing the subject: authorship, writing and the reader'. In: T. de Lauretis (ed.) *Feminist Studies/Critical Studies*. London: Macmillan, pp. 102–20.

Murphy E., Dingwall R., Greatbatch D., Parker S., Watson P. (1998) 'Qualitative research methods in health technology assessment: a review of the literature'. *Health Technology Assessment* 2: 16.

Oakley A., Olivers S., Peersman G. (1996) *Review of Effectiveness of Health Promotion Interventions for Men who have Sex with Men*. London: EPI Centre, London University Institute of Education.

Pawson N., Tilley R. (1997) *Realistic Evaluation*. London: Sage.

Peterson A., Bunton., R. (eds) (1997) *Foucault Health and Medicine*. London: Routledge.

Poland B. (1992) 'Learning to "walk our talk": the implications of sociological theory for research methodologies in health promotion'. *Canadian Journal of Public Health* 83 (Supplement 1), 531: 46.

Rosenau P. (1994) 'Health politics meets post-modernism: its meaning and implications for community health organising'. *Journal of Health Politics, Policy and Law* 19: 303–33.

Rubenstein L., Calkins D., Greenfield S., Jette A., Meenan R., Nevins M., Rubenstein L., Wasson J., Williams M. (1989) 'Health status assessment for elderly patients: report of the society of general internal medicine task force on health assessment'. *Journal of the American Geriatrics Society* 37: 562–9.

Sayer A. (1994) *Method in Social Science: A Realist Approach*. London: Hutchinson.

Stevenson H., Burke M. (1992) 'Bureaucratic logic in new social movement clothing; the limits of health promotion research'. *Canadian Journal of Public Health* 83 (Supplement 1): S47–S53.

Tones K., Tilford S. (1994) *Health Education: Effectiveness, Efficiency and Equity*. London: Chapman and Hall.

Usher R. (1996) 'Telling a story about research and research as story-telling: post-modern approaches to social research'. In: D. Avison *et al. Understanding Social Research: Perspectives on Methodology and Practice*. Southampton: University of Southampton.

Webb D. (1997) 'Measuring effectiveness in health promotion' (unpublished M.Sc. thesis). Southampton: University of Southampton.

—— (1999) 'Current approaches to gathering evidence'. In: D. Perkins, I. Simnett and L. Wright (eds) *Evidence-based Health Promotion*. Chichester: John Wiley and Sons.

World Health Organization (WHO) (1978) *Alma Ata 1978: Primary Health Care*. Geneva: WHO.

—— (1984) *Health Promotion: A Discussion Document on the Concepts and Principles*. Supplement to *Europe News* 3. Copenhagen: WHO.

—— (1986) *Ottawa Charter for Health Promotion*. Copenhagen: WHO.

Young I. (1990) *Justice and the Politics of Difference*. New Jersey: Princeton University Press.

—— (1995) 'The ideal of community and the politics of difference'. In: P. Weiss and M. Friedman (eds) *Feminism and Community*. London: Routledge, pp. 233–57.

Chapter 6

Evidence and the evaluation of a community-level intervention
Researching the Gay Men's Task Force initiative

Paul Flowers, Jamie Frankis and Graham Hart

Introduction

Evidence-based health promotion and particularly evidence-based *sexual* health promotion, have become goals to which researchers, commissioners and service providers alike aspire. Over the last few years much has been written and said about the need and value of such work, but little of this seems to have been put into practice (Hart 1996, Flowers 1997). However, several key questions have emerged which foster a healthy sense of reflexive inquiry for all those involved in both researching and delivering sexual health promoting services. What kind of evaluation should be adopted? What constitutes evidence of effectiveness? Which methodologies and designs are best suited to providing such evidence?

In this chapter we describe the design, implementation and monitoring of a single community-level intervention, the Gay Men's Task Force (GMTF) initiative, based in the gay bars of Glasgow, Scotland. The GMTF initiative is a community-level, community-based, inter-agency collaboration funded by Greater Glasgow Health Board and evaluated by the Gay Men's Sexual Health research team based in the MRC Social and Public Health Sciences Unit at the University of Glasgow. The initiative has three key components all independently shown to be effective in promoting sexual health amongst gay men, but which have never been combined previously (see Kegeles and Hart 1998). These are: peer education, a free telephone hotline and gay men specific sexual health projects based in both a hospital setting and an inner city

Gay and Lesbian Community Centre. The initiative began in October 1997 and was funded until June 1998. This chapter does not report empirical findings relating to the intervention itself but seeks to stimulate constructive discussion through a description of our experience of evaluating a specific intervention.

Here we illustrate the diverse ways in which the intervention was designed, monitored and will be evaluated. These evaluative methods are intended to capture much of the process by which the intervention is delivered and to determine its effectiveness through the use of pre-specified outcomes. Throughout, we employ a range of 'evidences', from so-called 'hard' measures, such as changes in behaviour (e.g. HIV testing rates, sexual health screening uptake), to 'soft' measures, such as the diaries of peer educators. This necessitates the adoption of a multi-method approach (including surveys and participant observation) encompassing different epistemological frameworks (positivism and phenomenology). We believe our broad-ranging approach to evidence-based sexual health promotion has particular strengths which should be shared and could be utilised by others.

The model of evaluation employed

Within the sexual health promotion field, Bonell (1996), among others, have highlighted the need for clarity in terms of the concepts and terminology used within intervention evaluation. Development work here describes the initial procedures of reviewing the relevant literature, searching for evidence of effectiveness, negotiating working relationships with other agencies (establishing healthy alliances) and other processes which consider issues of feasibility and appropriateness. We intend the 'formative evaluation' to reflect the on-going dialogue between researchers (evaluators) and intervention provision. It presents those feedback mechanisms which affect the intervention as it progresses. As Bonell writes, 'formative evaluations attempt to draw conclusions in order to refine the form of an intervention' (26). Process evaluation can be thought of as an examination of the 'activities involved in undertaking an intervention' (8), or as 'tracking the process of change occurring as a result of an intervention and identifying the factors that facilitate and constrain desired changes' (Wimbush, personal communication). Outcome evaluation, on the other hand, is concerned with assessing the effectiveness of an intervention by 'indicating whether an intervention has actually achieved its objectives in terms of the outcomes achieved' (20).

At each stage of the evaluation there has been a close partnership between researchers and intervention provision. Reflection on the intervention process from practitioners was welcomed by the researchers before and during the intervention. Regular meetings between representatives from each organisation involved with the Gay Men's Task Force were held to discuss the intervention and set the continuing agenda. It was at these meetings that the researchers presented the process evaluation (where appropriate) as the intervention progressed. There was also an on-going dialogue between researchers and service providers during the intervention on a less formal basis, where issues were discussed with the appropriate parties as they arose. It is the relationship between research and service provision that informs the structure of this chapter. Four key sections are presented which describe chronologically the complex interplay of research and intervention provision: developmental work, formative evaluation, process evaluation and outcome evaluation. Table 6.1 illustrates the evaluative processes employed at each of these stages (discussed more fully below).

Development work

Development work began with a literature review seeking to identify evidence of effectiveness in previous interventions among gay men. Working relationships between agencies began to be negotiated, existing and future service provision was assessed and we had the task of encouraging partners in this process to consider the potential value of research in sexual health service provision.

Throughout the 1990s, sex between men has been the primary cause of incident HIV infection in Scotland, with 74 per cent of new cases in this category. Since 1988 there has been a significant annual increase in the number of cases in this group (ANSWER 1995). It was clear that gay men in Scotland presented a particular population in which HIV risk behaviours were still occurring and that further prevention activity was needed. The highest number of cases of HIV infection in gay men in Scotland are to be found in Glasgow and Edinburgh. Given our interest in community-level interventions, these cities constituted ideal locations for the evaluation of novel sexual health interventions. The two cities are geographically close (only forty-five miles apart) yet have discrete

Table 6.1   Overview of research structure (1995–1999)

	Glasgow	Edinburgh
Development work	Literature review	
	Inter-agency negotiations	
Formative evaluation	Census	Census
	Participant observation	Participant observation
	Baseline data – survey	Baseline data – survey
	Focus groups	Focus groups
	Individual in-depth interviews	Individual in-depth interviews
Intervention	GMTF initiative and Existing services	Existing services
Process evaluation	Peer educators	
	Monitoring forms	
	Focus groups	
	Face-to-face interviews	
	Logging of hotline calls	
	GMTF agencies meetings	
Outcome evaluation	Outcome survey	Outcome survey
	Follow-up surveys	Follow-up surveys

cultural identities. Each city has a similar number of commercial gay venues, and similar numbers of men attending them. We therefore determined that some form of comparative study involving Glasgow and Edinburgh was potentially both feasible and desirable.

Outcome evaluations have been privileged as epistemologically superior to other forms of evaluative research in recent years, particularly those studies employing experimental research designs, with randomised controlled trials (RCTs) suggested as the gold standard by which to determine methodological rigour (Oakley *et al.* 1995). We identified evidence of effectiveness in a series of papers that had employed experimental or RCT designs. These suggested that amongst American gay men, peer-led, bar-based approaches were effective in reducing the incidence of unprotected anal intercourse (Kelly *et al.* 1991, 1992, 1997). There is also evidence that 'safer-sex hotlines' are effective in this respect (Coates *et al.* 1996).

This initial development work set a research agenda with clear questions relating to research design (e.g. are the gay men of Glasgow and Edinburgh comparable populations, and how much movement is there between the cities?), intervention method (are bar-based, peer-oriented approaches transferable from small American cities to large Scottish cities?) and intervention content (what are the specific sexual health needs of gay men in Glasgow?). These intervention implementation questions are best answered within what we describe as 'formative evaluation'.

Formative evaluation

Formative evaluation involves an on-going dialogue between research and intervention provision; it establishes the feedback mechanisms which directly affect the elements of an intervention and incorporates those processes which determine the feasibility and practicality of ideas suggested within earlier, developmental work. Formative evaluation is therefore concerned to operationalise intervention ideas and provide the research base for subsequent process and outcome evaluations.

Census and participant observation

It was necessary to ensure the feasibility of both researching and conducting an intervention within the gay bars of Glasgow. The existing literature suggested that gay bars were suitable places to access large numbers of men and, indeed, within gay men's sexual health research, response rates to questionnaires tend to be higher from bars than from other recruitment sites. For example, St Lawrence *et al.* (1989) report a response rate of 86 per cent in a bar study, contrasting sharply with 31 per cent of young gay men recruited from mainly non-bar sources (Hays *et al.* 1990). Bars also constitute a discrete social space, representing a distinct milieu (the 'scene') familiar to gay men themselves. The data generated by this approach may therefore be representative of a city's bar-going gay population (see Harry 1986 for a discussion of sampling gay men).

Over a one-week period we undertook a census of the number of men in gay bars and clubs in Glasgow, at two specific time periods (early and late evening) each day. Informal participant observation was also undertaken, assessing the ease with which men could be approached, and ease of audibility and visibility (to complete a questionnaire). Particular attention was paid to the movement of men within each venue. In the bars, for example, men remained relatively static, contrasting sharply to night-clubs which were filled with a highly mobile population of men moving from the dance floor to the bar and around the club. Audibility and light levels varied considerably between type of venue, with the clubs being very noisy, poorly lit and filled with people dancing and meeting sexual partners. In contrast, bars varied in degree of audibility but all were well lit, and although people were drinking and meeting sexual partners, there was a distinct culture of sociability. It was culturally appropriate for men to approach each other and begin conversations and we therefore surmised that men could be asked to complete self-administered questionnaires (SAQs). This approach was later repeated in Edinburgh and yielded similar conclusions.

We used a power calculation to determine the sample size required to measure a significant effect of the intervention. At the time of the formative evaluation, the earlier work of Kelly *et al.* (1991, 1992) represented the only studies detailing gay men's behaviour change after an intervention with a peer education element. The main outcome measure of both studies was a post-intervention reduction in the proportion of men reporting unprotected anal intercourse (UAI) in the previous two months (between 15 per cent and 37 per cent less than baseline (Kelly *et al.* 1991, 1992). In most studies of gay men's sexual behaviour, approximately one third of men report having engaged in UAI in the last year (Hart *et al.* 1993, Hickson *et al.* 1996, Hope and MacArthur 1998, Nardone *et al.* 1997), so we made a conservative estimate that 25 per cent of our sample would report some UAI in the previous year. Based on Kelly *et al.* (1991, 1992), we sought to reduce reported UAI by at least 20 per cent. We therefore, determined, using 80 per cent power, that we needed a minimum sample size of 1,133 in order to detect an intervention effect at the 95 per cent significance level. In Glasgow, the numbers counted in the census were sufficient (n = 2,616), even given the possibility of double counting, to meet this requirement. The Edinburgh census counted 2,085 men; again, given the possibility of double counting, this generated a likely sample size of 1,042. Therefore, assuming we could achieve a good response rate, in fourteen visits to Glasgow's and Edinburgh's five exclusively gay bars, we could expect to recruit enough men to measure likely intervention effects.

Baseline survey of gay men's behaviour

Whether Glasgow and Edinburgh could be used as intervention and control cities depended upon the comparability of gay populations in the two cities. Furthermore, the likely content of any given intervention had to be determined. With the rise in HIV seroconversion amongst gay men in Scotland, the reduction of UAI seemed prerequisite, yet the wider sexual health needs of gay men also had to be addressed. A short SAQ was developed and piloted. It requested a unique identifier (see below), demographic information, details of movement between Glasgow and Edinburgh, reported sexually transmitted infections (STIs), use of the commercial gay scene, perceptions of a safer sex culture and recent sexual behaviour.

This brief questionnaire was important for both formative and outcome evaluation. For the formative evaluation it demonstrated the relative ease of approaching men in gay bars (see response rate below). It also provided essential information relating to the movement of men between the cities, a demographic profile of gay men therein, and also an outline of key sexual health behavioural needs to be addressed within an intervention (i.e. an operational needs assessment). For the outcome evaluation it provided a measure of baseline sexual behaviour (see below).

With regard to the use of SAQs to provide measures of gay men's sexual behaviour, there are issues relating to the reliability and validity of these reports. Catania et al. (1990: 341) conclude that 'in general, sex research lacks a gold standard for validating self-reported sexual behaviour'. However, several studies suggest that self-reported sexual behaviour is reliable (Saltzman et al. 1987; Coates et al. 1986; Seage et al. 1992) though subject to the effects of recall period (Kauth et al. 1991; Coates et al. 1988) and content, with riskier behaviours less likely to be reported (Coates et al. 1988). In view of this, all data relating to HIV risk related behaviours must be viewed cautiously as representing an underestimate of the actual levels of risky sexual behaviour. Recall periods of both the previous month and the previous year were employed in the SAQ and data gathering within other parts of the intervention. Given the consistent use of recall periods and mode of data collection across the whole study, it is hoped that variability in men's reporting of sexual behaviour will be limited.

In February 1996 we made fourteen visits (every other day) to the gay bars of Glasgow, and in Edinburgh fourteen visits were made in November 1996. In Glasgow 1,245 of 1,619 men agreed to participate, and in Edinburgh 1,031 of 1,295 men who were approached participated. This gave a total of 2,276 men and a response rate of 78.5 per cent. The numbers of men already approached were also monitored across the fourteen visits; a steady increase in men already approached was observed, though saturation, in which all men present had already been approached, was never reached.

Table 6.2 presents the data collected in both Glasgow and Edinburgh through the SAQ. It demonstrates comparability between the cities in respect of sexual behaviour and social demographics. Of central importance is the low degree of movement between the two cities, with 88 per cent of Glasgow men and 87 per cent of Edinburgh men visiting the other city's gay scene fewer than seven times in the previous year. Thus there appears to be little scope for contamination by intervention effect between the two cities.

Exploratory research: the psychosocial context of sexual health and receptiveness to intervention ideas

A programme of qualitative research was undertaken to explore the social context of sexual behaviour and sexual health. In-depth interviews explored how men understood both the pursuit of sex and the meaning of sex itself in a variety of contexts. A semi-structured interview schedule highlighted several key areas to be discussed: men's perceptions of the commercial gay scene in Glasgow, the situations in which sex occurred, the situations in which unprotected sex occurred and the meanings of sexual activity. These data proved invaluable in designing a culturally appropriate peer education recruitment strategy (see Flowers and Hart 1998 for more details). A similar set of interviews is currently being conducted in Edinburgh.

Table 6.2   Demographic and recruitment characteristics

Description	Glasgow (n = 1,245) %	Edinburgh (n = 1,031) %	Total (n = 2,276) %
Age			
16–25	27	28	28
26–30	27	24	26
31–36	24	22	23
37 or older	22	26	24
Social class			
I and II	53	51	52
III N and III M	32	39	35
IV and V	15	11	13
Highest educational qualification			
Secondary	30	29	29
Further/vocational	33	32	33
Degree/post-grad. qualification	37	39	38
Area postcode			
Glasgow	71	4	41
Edinburgh	3	77	36
Rest of Scotland	21	12	17
Rest of UK	5	7	6
Visits to other city (in last year)			
None	51	48	50
1–6 times	37	39	38
7 plus times	12	14	13

Continued:

Description	Glasgow (n = 1,245) %	Edinburgh (n = 1,031) %	Total (n = 2,276) %
Frequency of visits to gay scene			
<1 per month	2	3	3
1 per month	11	12	11
2–3 per month	31	30	31
1–2 per week	40	42	41
4–5 per week	16	14	15
Sexual behaviour in the last year			
Number of partners			
None	3	2	3
One	21	21	21
2–	31	33	32
6 or more	45	45	45
Number of anal sex partners			
None	25	26	25
One	34	32	33
2–5	29	29	29
6 or more	13	13	13
Unprotected anal sex partners			
None	66	70	68
One	25	23	24
2–5	7	6	7
6 or more	2	1	1
Sexual history			p value (χ^2)
Lifetime history of STI	32	41	p<0.00001
STI in the last year	9	13	p<0.004
HIV antibody tested	47	55	p<0.0002

Note: STI = sexually transmitted infection

The in-depth interviews employed an inductive approach attempting to engage with the participant's view of his world. In contrast, focus groups were conducted in order to explicitly 'market test' ideas which had stemmed from the results of the baseline survey data collection (see Table 6.1). These were structured around ideas concerning the key elements of the proposed intervention. Partici-pants were drawn from existing community groups and were invited to participate if they were familiar with Glasgow's commercial gay scene. Thirty men from a variety of backgrounds took part in four focus group discussions, providing valuable insights into the likely community reception of these ideas.

Process evaluation: research and intervention

Here we use 'process evaluation' to refer to evaluation of the elements involved in the actual *delivery* of an intervention. This includes both the perspectives of those delivering and receiving services, in addition to the routine tasks of monitoring and audit. From its inception the Gay Men's Task Force was conceptualised as a peer-led community-level intervention. It was intended to have a community-wide effect, with an impact on many men, but only a fraction of those affected would necessarily have direct contact with the intervention itself. Therefore, the outcome evaluation seeks to measure aggregate community-wide changes in sexual health behaviour. In contrast, the process evaluation measures only those intervention aspects concerned with direct service provision to specific men – those who have primary contact with the intervention.

Unique identifier

We have attempted to employ a 'unique identifier' to follow individuals anonymously throughout the intervention. We requested each individual's date of birth, first part of their postcode and mother's maiden name initials which together provide a unique and robust identifier, enabling us to not only examine community-wide change in the outcome data collection (see below) but also track individuals throughout the intervention itself. For example, someone born on 21 October 1969, whose mother's maiden name was Mary Scott and who now resides in the Govanhill area of Glasgow (G42) would have this identifier: 211069G42MS. It was our hope that this information be requested in all client contacts. However, the local gay and lesbian switchboard which managed the freephone telephone hotline considered such a request to be inappropriate in an anonymous service, and therefore did not collect the information. Requests for unique identifier information within the initial survey (SAQ) were well received, with 90.4 per cent of all participants providing the necessary elements of the identifier. This was matched by the positive response of men in bars when approached by a peer educator; 94.8 per cent of participants have been willing to provide it. Similarly, 77.6 per cent of men using the clinical services in the intervention supplied this information.

Referral

Each time a participant comes into direct contact with the intervention, information regarding referral points is taken; men are asked how they had heard about a particular aspect of the intervention and from what source. In this way it becomes possible to calculate the efficacy of referral between intervention components; for example, the proportion of people using the telephone hotline who later attend the GUM services.

Experiential aspects of the intervention

A variety of qualitative methods has also been employed to examine the experiential aspects of the intervention itself. Diaries were provided to peer educators to record their own experiences, for which training was provided. It was intended that these should be a medium for peer educators to detail their perceptions of success and failure, the difficulties they face and the personal impact of working in bars and talking to gay men about sex, safer sex and sexual health. It was intended that this experiential element would inform the intervention, with modifications and improvements to it as it progressed. In future prevention initiatives, account could be taken of the views of the peer educators so that they could be better supported to deliver an improved service. However, little useful information resulted from the diaries, because peer educators, after spending several hours in gay bars, were too tired to complete their diaries. We are now relying on individual in-depth interviews and focus group discussions conducted with both peer educators and men active on the gay scene, in order to examine similar topics.

Routine monitoring

Multiple monitoring procedures provide on-going audit of each intervention element (i.e. peer educator interactions, telephone hotline and GUM services). These provide information on each individual interaction between service provider and service user. However, when linked through the unique identifier and referral system a secondary level of analysis is possible as the individual can be followed across multiple intervention exposures and indeed between intervention components.

With regard to the work of the peer educators, each interaction is recorded on a monitoring form. As well as requesting the information which constitutes the unique identifier and referral, the form assesses the overall content of each interaction by documenting the main sexual health and psychosocial health topics which have been discussed (from a wide ranging list of alternatives). This is done in two ways: three topics that the client has raised and three main topics that the peer educator has raised are recorded. Details of the duration and location of the interaction are also recorded (i.e. the bar in which the conversation took place), as are the identity of the peer educator (allowing analysis by educator and educator gender), the leaflets, if any, that were distributed and any additional comments the peer educator wishes to make.

The telephone hotline is also monitored, with each call logged according to the duration of the interaction and the three main sexual and psychosocial health topics which have been discussed (from a wide ranging list of alternatives). If the client is willing, brief demographic details are also taken and the destination of referral is also noted (e.g. to the peer educators in bars).

The clinical notes of an existing gay-men specific GUM project were adapted to be used within the GMTF initiative. Consent is sought that information may be passed on to the MRC (including details of the unique identifier so that individuals can be followed over multiple visits to the clinic). Each client provides demographic information, a sexual history for the preceding month and year (comparable to those used within the survey SAQ), a twelve-month recreational drug history and then, depending upon the kind of services received, details from health advisors, nursing staff, doctors and/or counsellors. Each element of the GUM service records the details of service provision (e.g. hepatitis B vaccination or domestic violence counselling), providing comprehensive documentation relating to each of a given client's visits to the services (both hospital- and gay and lesbian community centre-based).

In summary, the methods used here capture much of the intervention process through the use of both quantitative and qualitative methods. Details of all clients using each intervention element are maintained and updated. From this we can generate databases describing both demographic details and the intervention content. By employing the unique identifier and referral questions we will be able to focus upon interactions between intervention elements and track individuals across the study period, providing, for example, an indication of intervention dose per client. Diverse qualitative methods (diaries, focus group discussions and individual in-depth interviews) have been employed to record the experiences of peer educators and similar work will examine the clinical aspects of the intervention itself.

Outcome evaluation

Outcome evaluation has come to present the mainstay of intervention evaluation. By outcome evaluation we refer to that work involved in assessing an intervention's efficacy, both in the short and long term. The outcome evaluation seeks to address the impact of the intervention in terms of pre-specified behavioural outcomes. It may or may not focus upon whether these individuals have been in direct contact with elements of the intervention.

As discussed, the aim of the baseline survey was to provide a needs assessment and baseline measures of various sexual health related behaviours in both Glasgow and Edinburgh. The baseline survey suggested that there were few sexual behavioural or demographic differences between gay men in these two cities and hence that they represented suitable comparison populations. The intervention takes place in addition to existing services in Glasgow, whilst in Edinburgh existing services continue as usual. Post-intervention outcome surveys will be conducted in both cities to assess intervention effects. This allows us to assess whether any identified effects in Glasgow occurred over and above temporal and secular changes observed in Edinburgh. The relatively low levels of social mixing between men in these cities suggest that community-level changes occurring as a result of the intervention in Glasgow are unlikely to extend to ('contaminate') Edinburgh.

The six primary intervention outcomes we seek are: a reduction in the rate of unprotected anal intercourse with casual partners in the previous year; an increase in the proportion of men reducing risk within relationships; for those men who practise 'negotiated safety' (see below), an increase in the proportion who know their own and their partner's HIV status; an increase in the proportion of men vaccinated against hepatitis B; and an increase in the proportion of men who know their HIV status based on a test. Secondary outcome measures have been specified through clinical audit: an increase in the numbers of men using the GUM services; an increase in the numbers of men completing a course of three hepatitis B vaccinations; and an increase in the numbers of men tested for HIV. These can be assessed both in terms of specific services dedicated to gay men in Glasgow as well as across all GUM services in the area served by the Greater Glasgow Health Board. It is difficult to specify the direction of post-intervention change, if any, in the proportion of gay men presenting at GUM services with acute STIs (including HIV, hepatitis B, gonorrhoea, syphilis, first attack genital warts and genital herpes). Clearly a decrease in the proportion of men presenting with these infections is desirable; however, an *increase* in this figure could represent a positive public health outcome if men self-refer to services because of increased awareness of sexual health. Infections would be treated earlier and aggregate transmission rates would therefore decrease.

Reported unprotected anal intercourse in the last year

Our initial power calculation, to determine sample size, was based on Kelly *et al.*'s observed change in reported UAI following a peer-education based intervention similar to ours. However, we do not consider that a reduction in reports of *any* UAI is an appropriate measure of intervention effectiveness. Though the majority of gay men have reduced their risk of HIV infection through consistent condom use (Hart *et al.* in press), other responses ('sexual strategies') have been adopted (cf. Schilts and Adam 1995) and are currently being promoted both within the gay community and by service providers (Hickson and Maguire 1996). For example, Kippax *et al.* (1993) discuss 'negotiated safety': not using condoms within a relationship is 'safe' if both men are HIV seronegative and have an explicit agreement concerning sex outwith their relationship, i.e. that any sex outside the relationship is 'safe' (for example no UAI with casual partners). There is evidence to show that 'the adoption of negotiated safety among men in HIV-seronegative regular relationships may help such men sustain the safety of their sexual practice' (Kippax *et al.* 1997: 191).

Clearly, rather than seeking a decrease in reported UAI *per se,* as did Kelly *et al.* (1991, 1992, 1997), we needed to distinguish those men in our population reporting UAI within what appears to be a safer-sexual strategy (i.e. akin to negotiated safety) from those reporting some UAI with casual partners. Successful intervention effects would include: an increase in men who report practising negotiated safety and/or a decrease in reported UAI with casual partners. The following calculations are based on a comparison of 1,031 subjects at baseline and post-intervention, with 80 per cent power to detect significant change (at the 95 per cent level).

REDUCTION IN UAI WITH CASUAL PARTNERS

Subsequent to the execution of our baseline survey, Kegeles *et al.* (1996) reported a 45 per cent reduction in reported UAI in the previous two months *with non-primary partners* from baseline levels of 20.2 per cent to 11.1 per cent. In our Glasgow sample, 39 per cent of men reported some UAI with *casual partners in the last year.* Our study will be able to detect a 15.5 per cent reduction in post-intervention reports of UAI with casual partners.

SAFER SEXUAL STRATEGIES WITH REGULAR PARTNERS

Very strict criteria were applied to identify men in our sample who were likely to be practising a 'negotiated safety' strategy. This group of men reported that when they practised UAI in the last year, this was always with a regular partner, that they always knew their partner's status, and that this partner was not HIV positive. These criteria excluded positive couples because of the risk of reinfection with drug resistant strains of HIV, and did not assess whether this was an explicit (openly discussed and agreed) strategy. It otherwise covered the essence of 'negotiated safety'. Of the Glasgow sample, 4 per cent fitted these criteria. The study would detect an increase of at least 72.5 per cent employing this strategy.

KNOWLEDGE OF OWN AND PARTNER'S STATUS

Men who report practising UAI with regular partners only may well be practising 'negotiated safety', but to do so successfully must know their own and their partner's HIV status. In our baseline survey, 332 Glasgow men (15 per cent of the sample) reported practising UAI with regular partners only. Of this sub-sample, 74.7 per cent reported that they knew their own HIV status, and 70.7 per cent reported that they knew their *partner's* HIV status. Assuming we achieve similar or greater numbers of men reporting UAI, with regular partners only, in the post-intervention survey, our study will be in a position to measure an increase of 12 per cent in the proportion of men in this sub-sample reporting that they know their own HIV status and an increase of 14 per cent of those who report knowledge of their partner's HIV status.

INCREASE IN HEPATITIS B VACCINATION RATES

In Glasgow 44 per cent of the men and in Edinburgh 53 per cent of the men reported being vaccinated against hepatitis B, a significant difference (χ^2 = 18.68, p<0.00003). The Glasgow rate marks only a slight increase over men surveyed in England over seven years ago (Hart *et al.* 1993) although is 10 per cent higher than for men in the West Midlands of England (Hope, personal communication). However, since gay men are one of the main groups at risk of hepatitis B and for them the vaccination is freely available, our finding still represents a low rate. A pressing aim of the GMTF intervention was to increase the proportion of men completing a course of three hepatitis B vaccinations. The study has the power to detect a 15 per cent change, which would represent 50.5 per cent of our post-intervention, Glasgow sample reporting vaccination.

INCREASE IN HIV TESTING RATES

Significantly fewer men in Glasgow (47 per cent) reported ever having had an HIV test compared to Edinburgh men (55 per cent) (χ^2 = 14.1, p<0.0002). These rates are much lower than men in London (Nardone *et al.* 1997), where 73 per cent of a non-clinical sample report ever having had an HIV test, and Australia, where most gay men in samples from Sydney (90.8 per cent), Melbourne (89.1 per cent) and Brisbane (86.6 per cent) know their status based on a test (Prestage *et al.* 1997). Our intervention aim is to increase the proportion of men who know their serostatus based on an HIV-antibody test. Our sample size will allow us to detect an increase of 13 per cent, or post-intervention a rate of 53.25 per cent of Glasgow men reporting an HIV test.

In summary, the outcome evaluation determines the effectiveness of the intervention at a community, as opposed to individual, level. Pre- and post-intervention questionnaires in Glasgow allow intervention effects to be measured, whilst the same surveys administered in Edinburgh allow any temporal effects to be controlled for. Primary outcomes of the intervention were specified *a priori*, concerning changes in sexual behaviours, sexual health vaccination and screening. We have discussed the level of change we will be able to detect, given a post-intervention sample at least as large at that achieved at baseline. In addition to this, the success of the intervention can also be measured at a clinical level, assessing long-term changes in the numbers of gay men attending general and gay-men specific GUM services in Glasgow, and their uptake of hepatitis B and HIV testing.

Discussion

In this chapter we have illustrated the complexity of evaluating a novel community-level intervention (the Gay Men's Task Force). The many evaluative methods we have employed have been organised into four key sections: development work, formative evaluation, process evaluation and outcome evaluation. The work discussed within the development section describes the groundwork which had to be done in selecting the most appropriate type of intervention (from the previous literature). The section relating to formative evaluation provided an outline of the feedback processes which operationalised the intervention, through a census and, to ensure cultural appropriateness, the use of qualitative methodologies (i.e. participant observation, in-depth interviews, focus groups). With regard to the process evaluation, we set in place monitoring procedures across the various intervention elements which, on a regular basis, record varying aspects of service delivery ranging from the routine audit of clinical procedures within GUM services to recording each peer education interaction within the bars. The outcome evaluation assesses potential intervention effects on several key outcome measures. Power calculations provided the level of change our sample size has 80 per cent power to detect, for each of the primary outcome measures. These are based on relative changes between pre- and post-intervention questionnaires in Glasgow, allowing us to control for temporal changes using data from repeat surveys in Edinburgh.

Our approach has been one of methodological pluralism in the face of the varied research questions posed by our evaluation design (Table 6.1). It is worth making explicit the reason behind the current interest in evaluating interventions. Given the urgency of a continuing HIV epidemic amongst gay men, limited resources should be targeted to where they are needed most and used in ways that are known to promote sexual health and reduce new HIV infections. This necessitates the use of experimental research designs which seek to establish effectiveness and highlights the role of cumulative knowledge through previous studies. However, it is not intervention effectiveness *per se*, we believe, that should be used to determine resource allocation or policy decisions but instead intervention utility (i.e. a demonstration of efficacy, transferability and sustainability). In this way, it is the long-term history of a given intervention's efficacy that is important, as it must be tried and tested in differing circumstances before the expense and effort of experimental evaluation can be dispensed with. Within this longer term view, the importance of differing types of intervention evaluation clearly changes; outcome evaluation is initially of primary concern. Subsequently, and given the key questions of transferability and sustainability, process and formative evaluation become more relevant as a record of how an intervention is operationalised and implemented. In this way, the utility of an intervention should not be decided only through a demonstration of effectiveness using outcome measures. Instead, a record of the intervention process and formative evaluation are essential in understanding the practicalities of transferability and gauging the likelihood of sustainability.

This chapter has provided an example of the various evaluative methods that we have employed in evaluating a specific peer-led community-level intervention. The rigour we have sought to apply to each step of evaluation (development, formative, process and outcome) reflects our commitment to evidence-based sexual health promotion, both by determining the efficacy of interventions, and more importantly, assessing the utility of an intervention in the long term. Although these diverse methods have been adopted in relation to the Gay Men's Task Force, they do represent a useful framework for other similar community-level interventions. Relatively simple procedures such as the unique identifier can be adopted and assimilated into routine monitoring and audit in situations where clients do not wish to provide names and addresses, and provides a more comprehensive record of service delivery, for example, distinguishing between number of clients and number of contacts (which may include repeat contacts). The self-complete questionnaires on sexual behaviour used in bars were very acceptable to gay men, and would probably be similarly successful if used with young heterosexual men and women in bars and clubs – thus extending the research base on sexual behaviour from its current, somewhat limited, spheres and formats.

Both the proponents and opponents of experimental methods in community-based intervention research, particularly randomised controlled trials, often fail to recognise the need for very different research methods to answer quite different research questions at each stage of the evaluation of a novel health-promotion intervention. This apparently self-evident truth is so often ignored in favour of a rhetoric of research superiority or hierarchy which is proposed by people who are determined to press the case for their chosen approach. We seek to combine research methods at each stage of the evaluation process, but also recognise that in order to understand *process* we must employ certain approaches, and that to understand *outcome* other measures are necessary. It is our view that epistemological and ideological boundaries must be crossed and indeed broken down if we are to have a research-based health promotion which achieves demonstrable health gain in the communities we serve.

Acknowledgements

This research is supported by the UK Medical Research Council and Greater Glasgow Health Board. Our thanks to staff of the Steve Retson Project, PHACE West, and Gay Switchboard for their collaboration in this study. We also wish to thank Leigh Harkin and Geoff Der for statistical support. Claire Marriott for her hard work and Erica Wimbush and Vivian Hope for their assistance.

References

ANSWER (1995, 1996): *HIV in Scotland: Annual Review to 31 December*, AM–19, no. 96/04.

Bonell C. (1996) *Outcomes in HIV prevention: Report of a Research Project*. London: The HIV Project.

Catania J., Gibson D., Chitwood D., Coates T. (1990) 'Methodological problems in AIDS behavioural research: influences on measurement error and participation bias in studies of sexual behaviour'. *Psychological Bulletin* 108: 339–62.

Coates R., Soskolne C., Calzavara L., Read S., Fanning M., Shepherd F., Klein M., Johnson J. (1986) 'The reliability of sexual histories in AIDS-related research: evaluation of an interview administered questionnaire'. *Canadian Journal of Public Health* 77: 343–8.

Coates R., Calzavara L., Soskolne C., Read S., Fanning M., Shepherd F., Klein M., Johnson J. (1988) 'Validity of sexual histories in a prospective study of male sexual contacts of men with AIDS or an AIDS related condition'. *American Journal of Epidemiology* 128: 19–28.

Coates T., Aggleton P., Gutzwiller F., Des Jarlais D., Kilhara M., Kippax S., Schechter M., van den Hoeck J. (1996) 'HIV prevention in developed countries'. *Lancet* 348: 1,143–8.

Flowers P., Sheeran P., Beail N., Smith, J. (1997) 'The role of psychosocial factors in HIV risk-reduction among gay and bisexual men: a quantitative review'. *Psychology and Health* 12: 197–230.

Flowers P. (1997) 'Interventions – gay men'. *Aids Care* 9: 57–62.

Flowers, P., Hart, G. (1998) 'Everyone on the scene is so cliquey: Are gay bars an appropriate social context for a community-based peer led intervention?' In: *AIDS: Family, Culture and Community*. London: Taylor & Francis.

Fullerton D., Holland J., Oakley A. (1995) 'Towards effective intervention: evaluating HIV prevention and sexual health education interventions'. In: P. Davies, G. Hart (eds) *AIDS, Safety, Sexuality and Risk*. London: Taylor & Francis.

Hart G., Flowers P., Der G., Frankis J. (in press) 'Gay men's HIV-related sexual risk behaviour in Scotland'. *Sexually Transmitted Infections*.

Hart G. (1996) 'Hope for evidence-based HIV/AIDS prevention?' *AIDS* 10: 337–8

Hart G., Dawson J., Fitzpatrick R., Boulton M., McLean L., Brookes M., Parry J. (1993) 'Risk behaviour, anti HIV and anti HBc prevalence in clinic and non-clinic samples of gay men in England 1991–2'. *AIDS* 7: 863–9.

Harry J. (1986) 'Sampling gay men'. *Journal of Sex Research* 22: 1–34.

Hays R., Kegeles S., Coates T. (1990) 'High HIV risk taking among young gay men'. *AIDS* 4: 901–7.

Hickson F., Maguire M. (1996) '*Thinking It Through* – a Booklet for Gay Men. Building Bridges conference, linking research and primary HIV prevention'. London: Institute of Education (8–9 March).

Hickson F., Reid D., Davies P., Weatherburn P., Beardsell S., Keogh P. (1996) 'No aggregate change in homosexual HIV risk behaviour among gay men attending the Gay Pride festivals, United Kingdom, 1993–1995'. *AIDS* 10: 771–4.

Hope V., MacArthur C. (1998) 'Safer sex and social class: findings from a study of men using the "gay scene" in the West Midlands Region of the United Kingdom'. *AIDS Care* 10: 81 – 8.

Kauth M., St. Lawrence J., Kelly J. (1991) 'Reliability of retrospective assessments of sexual HIV-risk behaviour. A comparison of biweekly, three month and 12 month self-reports'. *AIDS Education and Prevention* 3: 207–14.

Kegeles S., Hart G. (1998) 'Recent HIV prevention interventions for gay men: individual, small-group and community-based studies'. *AIDS* (in press).

Kegeles S., Hays R., Coates T. (1996) 'The Mpowerment project: a community-level HIV prevention intervention for young gay men'. *American Journal of Public Health* 86: 1,129–36.

Kelly J., St.Lawrence J., Diaz Y., Stevenson L., Hauth A., Kalichman S., Brasfield T., Smith J., Andrew M. (1991) 'HIV risk-related behaviour reduction following intervention with key opinion leaders of population: an experimental analysis'. *American Journal of Public Health* 81: 168–71.

Kelly J., St.Lawrence J., Stevenson L., Hauth A., Kalichman S., Diaz Y., Brasfield T., Koob J., Morgan M. (1992) 'Community AIDS/HIV risk-reduction: the effects of endorsements by popular people in three cities'. *American Journal of Public Health* 82: 1,483–9.

Kelly J., Murphy D., Sikkema K., McAuliffe T., Roffman R., Solomon L., Winett R., Kalichman S. and the Community HIV Prevention Research Collaborative (1997) 'Randomised, controlled, community-level HIV-prevention intervention for sexual-risk behaviour among homosexual men in US cities'. *Lancet* 350: 1,500–5.

Kippax S., Noble J., Prestage G., Crawford J., Campbell D., Baxter D., Cooper D. (1997) 'Sexual negotiation in the AIDS era: negotiated safety revisited'. *AIDS* 11: 191–7.

Kippax S., Crawford J., Davis M., Rodden P., Dowsett G. (1993) 'Sustaining safe sex: a longitudinal study of a sample of homosexual men'. *AIDS* 7: 257–63.

Nardone A., Mercey D., Johnson A. (1997) 'Surveillance of sexual behaviour among homosexual men in a central London health authority'. *Genitourinary Medicine* 73: 198–202.

Oakley A., Fullerton D., Holland J. (1995) 'Behavioural interventions for HIV/AIDS prevention'. *AIDS* 9: 479–86.

Prestage G., Knox S., Kippax S., Benton K., Mahat M., Crawford J., Richters J., French J., Van de Ven P. (1997) *A Demographic and Behavioural Comparison of Three Samples of Homosexually Active Men in Sydney, Melbourne and Brisbane.* Report by National Centre in HIV Social Sciences, School of Behavioural Sciences, Macquarie University, Sydney NSW 2109, Australia.

Saltzman S., Stoddard A., McCusker J., Moon M., Mayer K. (1987) 'Reliability of self-reported sexual behaviour risk factors for HIV infection in homosexual men'. *Public Health Reports* 102: 692–7.

Schilts M.-A., Adam P. (1995) 'Reputedly effective risk education strategies and gay men'. In P. Aggleton, P. Davies, G. Hart (eds) *AIDS: Safety, Sexuality and Risk.* London: Taylor & Francis.

Seage G., Mayer K., Horsburgh C., Cal B., Lamb G. (1992) 'Corroboration of sexual histories among male homosexual couples'. *American Journal of Epidemiology* 135: 79–84.

St. Lawrence J., Hood H., Brasfield T., Kelly J. (1989) 'Differences in gay men's AIDS risk knowledge and behaviour patterns in high and low AIDS prevalence cities'. *Public Health Reports* 104: 391–5.

Smith J. (1996) 'Beyond the divide between cognition and discourse: using interpretative phenomenological analysis in health psychology'. *Psychology and Health* 11: 261–71.

Wight D. *Using Qualitative Research in a Randomised Controlled Trial of Sex Education.* Joint MRC/ESRC meeting on health behavioural interventions. 30 April–1 May 1997.

Chapter 7

Implementation of health promotion policy in Norwegian municipalities

Elisabeth Fosse

Introduction

Norway has a population of approximately 4.5 million people. There are 435 municipalities, most of which are relatively small. Two-hundred-and-forty-seven have less than 5,000 inhabitants, and only nine have more than 50,000 inhabitants. On the other hand, more than 1.2 million people live in the nine largest municipalities, while a little less than 650,000 live in the smallest ones (*Kommunenøkkelen* 1996). In common with other Scandinavian countries, Norway has a large public sector.

From the 1970s there has been a general tendency towards decentralisation throughout the Western world. Decentralisation reforms have been a vehicle for modernisation especially to make public administration more efficient. Decentralisation is expected to be a solution to problems of flexibility and accountability (Rouban 1993).

Norwegian central and local government

The expansion of the Nordic welfare states has, over the last decades, primarily taken place at the local level. Local authorities have been responsible for the implementation of welfare state programmes. The Norwegian policy has been called 'modernisation through decentralisation'. In an international context, the Nordic countries are said to stand firmly on local feet (Baldersheim and Ståhlberg 1994). Today, there are roughly twice as many employees in local authorities as there were twenty-five years ago. Public consumption in 1992 at the local level was 59 per cent in Norway, 69 per cent in Denmark and 71 per cent in Sweden. In Germany it is 17 per cent and in Britain 36 per cent (Fimreite and Ryssevik 1998).[1]

Local authorities have, for a number of reasons, been at the centre of national reforms in Norwegian government (Baldersheim and Ståhlberg 1994). Local authorities are small scale and are close to citizens. In many ways, local authorities represent civic society. For the welfare state local authorities have the additional advantage of being at the bottom level of a hierarchical governing system.

Until 1986, Norwegian municipalities were financed by earmarked grants. In 1986 the financing system was changed into economic grants which, in principle, granted local authorities the opportunity to decide how the grants were to be spent. The three most important municipal sectors are education, health and social services.[2] Approximately two-thirds of municipal expenses are tied to services within these sectors (Fimreite and Ryssevik 1998).[3]

The relationship between national and local authorities has altered as a consequence of changes in the income system and other decentralisation policies. These reforms require different ways of interacting between administrative levels. As a consequence of the decentralisation reforms, national government has devolved authority towards the local level.

The former government system was a prescriptive and top down system, based on earmarked funding. The governing tools were characterised as 'carrot and whip'. In a decentralised system, however, mostly 'soft' governing tools are available for central government. Information is one such tool. Another is time-limited programmes, where national government funds actions and interventions in municipalities for a limited period of time, to stimulate municipalities to take on certain policies and actions. The most extensive experiment of this kind was the Free Commune Programme in the late 1980s. Another is the programme discussed in this chapter, The National Programme for Health Promotion (subsequently referred to as the Programme).

Health promotion policy in a Norwegian context

After the Second World War, a strong centralised health administration was built up in Norway. It consisted of administrations at the central, regional and local levels. The National Board of Health[4] (the Board) came to play a dominant part in Norwegian health policy, especially under its leader from 1945 to 1972, Karl Evang. This was the period of the building of the social-democratic welfare state. Priority was given to the building of hospitals and the improvement and development of the medical care system. The primary health care system was a hierarchy that consisted of the National Board of Health, the County Medical Officers and the Local Medical Officers. The medical profession held a dominant position in this system, both as medical experts and as administrators. The period from 1945 until the 1970s has been called the period of 'professiocracy' in Norwegian health administration (Nordby 1987).

This was changed during the 1980s and 1990s, for various reasons. One was the desire for more political control over the Board (Christensen 1994). This resulted in two reorganisations, in both of which the authority of the Board was weakened. The first took place in 1983, and it resulted in a division of the Board. Part of its administration was placed as a department within the Ministry of Health and Social Affairs (the Ministry). The process of the second reorganisation took place during the period of the National Programme, from 1992 to 1993. In this reorganisation the National Board of Health lost the rest of its independence. The reorganisation placed the Board entirely as a subordinate institution under the Ministry.

Parallel to these reorganisations, the ideology of decentralisation was growing more dominant. The centralised, state dominated Board of Health no longer fitted into a model of decentralised, locally organised health services. The Act of Municipal Health Services in Norway was implemented in 1984. The Act was part of the political decentralisation process, in the sense that municipalities were given the political and administrative responsibility for primary health care. In the Act, health promotion was given high priority. This was further underlined in 1988 when two clauses were added to the Municipal Health Act. One stated that health promotion was a field of intersectoral responsibility, the other made municipalities responsible for environmental health.

An evaluation of the Municipal Health Act was carried out in 1989. It showed that the field of health promotion had a smaller growth than the other fields of the health services (Stortingsmelding nr. 6 1989–9).

In the 1990s, the priority given to health promotion has been further underlined. This is reflected in Government White Papers concerning the 'Health For All' strategies and the 'Ottawa Charter'. Both strategies have been included in Norwegian health policy (Stortingsmelding nr. 41 1987–88, Stortingsmelding nr. 37 1992–93).

In government documents, the Ottawa Charter is outlined as the basis for health promotion policy. This implies that health promotion has a wider scope and a different ideology from that of disease prevention. More specifically, health promotion involves many aspects of municipal activity and covers all sectors, while disease prevention is a matter for the health services. In health promotion, the focus is on living conditions, and ideally involves a critical focus on policy, communities and professions (Jensen 1983). Disease prevention, on the other hand, deals with the traditional tasks of the health services. In health promotion, intersectoral co-operation is central. This is also stressed in the Government White Papers. In disease prevention, however, it is the classical role of the professions as experts that is being underlined. Compliance with the advice of the experts will thus be important (Rimpelä 1984).

In the present study, the focus is on the implementation of The National Programme for Health Promotion. The points of departure for the Programme were the 'new' ideologies of health promotion, as stated in the Ottawa Charter and in the Government White Papers. The objectives of the Programme were to contribute to an increased focus on health promotion in the municipalities and to stimulate more intersectoral co-operation. Nevertheless, the local health services were given administrative responsibility for the projects. According to the arguments above, this might seem contradictory, in terms of implementing health promotion policy, since the health sector has focused mainly on disease prevention.

Theoretical framework

In the theoretical approaches to implementation studies, two main foci have been outlined. These approaches have usually been called 'top down' and 'bottom up' (Elmore 1979, 1985), and in recent years, the *decision perspective* and the *process perspective*. These latter are the concepts used in this chapter (Kjellberg and Reitan 1995).

The point of departure in a decision perspective is 'the legal imperative'. This implies that the statutory decision is a basis for studying the implementation process. Research questions will be focused on whether or not the policies were implemented according to stated intentions. As a consequence of this, mainly organisational variables have been studied. In the literature a primary focus has been on the content of the policy. If a policy that is going to be implemented is likely to result in minor change and there is consensus about it, it is likely to be implemented. However, if the policy represents major change, and there is conflict about it, it is more likely that it will not be implemented (van Meter and van Horn 1975, Mazmanian and Sabatier 1981, Sabatier 1986).

In the process perspective, the implementation is studied mainly as an empirical process. The process is studied independently of the objectives of the policy. In this perspective, the cognitions and actions of the actors who participate in the implementation process are the central focus of research (Hjern 1982, Hjern and Hull 1982).

Traditionally, the decision perspective and the process perspective have been considered contradictory. During the last years, however, several authors have argued for a combination of perspectives (Elmore 1985, Castongs and Springett 1997, Pawson and Tilley 1997).

In this setting the strongest arguments for a combination of the decision perspective and the process perspective concerns the objectives of the Programme, which is a means of implementing the Municipal Health Act. National Acts are the strongest form of legitimacy in democratic countries. On this basis, it is relevant whether or not the objectives of the Programme were achieved or not. On the other hand, the Programme is a 'soft' governing tool and much authority is given to the municipalities in shaping and carrying out the projects. One of the aims of such Programmes will be to learn through experiences built up during the process. In this setting, it will also be of significance to try and understand the role of the local actors in the process.

In the present study, the two approaches have been combined. They each give answers to different research questions. While the decision perspective can provide answers to *what* happened and *how* it happened, the process perspective can provide answers to *why* it happened. This is illustrated in Table 7.1.

Table 7.1   Research focus in a decision perspective and a process perspective on implementation

Research questions	Theoretical approach	Implementation
What?/How?	Decision perspective	Role of/change in organisations
Why?	Process perspective	Role of/change in actors

In implementation theory the main focus is on the process after a policy has been formulated and decided upon. However, the policy-formulation process constitutes the framework for the policy. This will always have effects on the implementation (Pressmann and Wildavsky 1973, Mazmanian and Sabatier 1981, Winter 1990). This is the rationale for choosing the central level also as a focus for the study.

Methods

The data considered in this chapter consisted of interviews and documents. The Programme under study lasted for five years, and the process was followed for most of the period. The state level is represented by the bodies that were in charge of the Programme, the Ministry of Health and Social Affairs and the National Board of Health. At the state level, all those who were involved in the Programme were interviewed. Data were collected twice, once early in the Programme and once after the Programme was over. Thirty-four persons were interviewed. The institutions that were represented were The Ministry of Health and Social Affairs, The National Board of Health, The Ministry of Environment,[5] The National Association of Local Authorities and the County Medical Officers.

Approximately 270 local projects were funded by the Programme. Five municipalities took part in the present study. The main criterion for choosing municipalities were the ideologies of the local projects, on the basis that they should not deal with traditional health sector tasks. Intersectoral co-operation should be central. All municipalities that took part in the study also had previous experience with the theme of the project.

One of the projects was not administered by the health services and is not discussed further in this chapter. The other four projects could be placed in two main groups, according to the fields they were working in. Two of them were *community-oriented* projects and two were dealing with *environment health* problems.[6]

In choosing the interviewees, I was looking for the 'implementation structures', i.e. the actors who took part in the implementation. The concept of implementation structures implies that there will be actors from different organisations who take part in the implementation process. The concept is an analytical one, and its focus is on actors rather than on organisations (Milward 1982, Hjern and Porter 1981).

Those interviewed were persons participating or co-operating with the projects, as well as political and administrative leaders. They were a fairly heterogeneous group, and generally the implementation structures were different in the community projects from those in the environment projects. The community projects focused on the people within communities and the projects dealt with interventions at the community level. The target group was mostly lay people. The environment projects, however, were more focused on local government and on the institutionalisation of the projects. The target group was mostly civil servants in the local authorities.

Eighty-nine people were interviewed in the municipalities. Data were collected three times, the last time after the Programme was ended. The interviews were semi-structured. The focus in the interviews was on how the projects were implemented, but also on the processes that could explain both why certain events took place and differences in implementation between the municipalities.

Further focus was on *actions* and *ideologies* in the projects. Among the topics that were raised were the content of the projects, with whom the projects were collaborating, and their relations with other sectors and the leadership in the municipalities. The actors' ideologies concerning health promotion and disease prevention and their attitudes to intersectoral co-operation were also explored. Both official documents concerning the projects and unofficial documents, e.g. memos and reports, were consulted.

According to Huberman and Miles (1994), the phase of data analysis is similar in quantitative and qualitative research. In both approaches the material will have to be sifted and reorganised in order to create meaning. In the present study, data were analysed according to the themes of the interview guide, and the two main topics, actions and ideologies. The analysis was conducted after each data collection and it was revised as the process in the projects changed and developed. As there was opportunity to follow the projects for most of the Programme period, it was possible to document outcomes as well as processes.

Empirical findings

State level

The Ministry and the Board were the central institutions at the state level. The Ministry had delegated the responsibility for the Programme to the Board. In a memo written in the initial phase of the Programme the Board focused on the need to strengthen the health administration at the central and the county level (Helsedirektoratet 1989: 22):

> The Programme ... will require 15 new and changed posts at the central and county level. ... It will be important for a future organisation that the County Medical Officers are active participants ... at the central level, the National Board of Health should have the main responsibility in co-ordinating and governing the main project.

In the opinion of the Board, it was the health sector that was going to be strengthened. Employees in the Board emphasised that the health sector should have a co-ordinating and supervising role in health promotion. One of the project leaders expressed it in the following way in an interview: 'We wanted to focus on the health services and what they could do. It was their experiences that were important to us. After all, the projects were organised by the health services.' The Ministry thought differently. The Director of the Department of Health Promotion felt that the good thing about the Programme was that the local authorities had the responsibility: 'The aim of the Programme is to start creative processes in the municipalities. ... It is important that the projects have strategies for co-operation and co-ordination.' The Director believed that the health sector should play a modest role in the projects and in health promotion in general: 'The most important actors in the municipalities are the political and administrative leadership. The health services don't have so much to offer in this kind of health promotion.'

These quotations demonstrate that ideologies were different in the Ministry and the Board. The Board understood health promotion more in line with the concept of disease prevention. This implies that the health services should play a dominant part in health promotion and have the role as *controller*. The Ministry, on the other hand, had an understanding more in line with WHO's concept of health promotion. This would imply that the health sector should be one among several equal actors in the field with a role as *co-worker*. The roles of the Ministry and the Board are illustrated in Table 7.2.

Figure 7.2.   Ideologies and strategies at the central level

Institutions	Strategies
Ministry of Health and Social Affairs	WHO-based strategies
	Ideology of health promotion
	Health sector as co-worker
The National Board of Health	Medical-oriented strategies
	Ideology of disease prevention
	Health sector as controller

As the Board had the administrative responsibility for the Programme, their strategy came to be dominant. The role of the Board might be viewed as a strategy for regaining its declining position. This, however, did not succeed. In 1993, the second reorganisation of the Health Administration was implemented. As pointed out previously, the consequence of this reorganisation was that the Board lost its independent position.

Municipal level

Previously, the four projects in this study were categorised in two types, community projects and environment projects. The two types reflect the 'new' fields of health promotion. They are fields which are not a traditional part of the health services and which require intersectoral co-operation. Still, there are marked differences between the two types of projects. The themes of the community projects are on the borderline between public and civic sectors. The target group is the population in the communities. The tasks are vague and have no distinct borders. The environment projects are different.[7] The field is institutionalised as a part of public sector. The target group for contact will mostly be civil servants and politicians. The field has got relatively distinct borders. In the present study, the community projects took place in peripheral rural municipalities, while the environment projects took place in central urban municipalities.

The community projects

As pointed out above, the community projects took place in rural municipalities in the periphery. In both communities fisheries were the dominant industry. Both had experienced problems in their industries, and in both the population was declining. In each municipality the projects took local problems as their point of departure. At the time of the projects, the problems had not been considered very closely by the local authorities and there had been little political debate on the issues.

In one of the municipalities, the point of departure was a crisis in the fisheries in the early 1990s. The shares the fishermen were allowed to catch were drastically reduced, and this led to unemployment and insecurity about the future. In the project, these problems were defined as health problems. It was suggested that the health sector should be consulted in these matters. In a letter that was distributed by the health services to all inhabitants this was expressed as follows:

> The crisis in the fisheries is also a health problem. The project has therefore decided that one public health nurse and one doctor will be persons to contact when an economic crisis turns up. The public health nurse and the doctor will primarily be a link between those who need help and those who can help them. The professional secrecy of the health services will make it easier for people to talk about economic and human problems created by the crisis in the fisheries.

The health services intended to contact other municipal sectors and even banks in order to help people. However, this strategy created problems for intersectoral co-operation. The social welfare sector naturally had a large increase in applications for social welfare at this time. Employees at the social welfare office reacted negatively to the assumption that it was easier to contact the health services than the social welfare office:

> The health services claimed that there was such a high threshold to the social welfare office. I don't think this was true, it was an external reason why people got problems. ... The social welfare office nearly drowned in new applications, due to the crisis in the fisheries.

The topic of the project concerned several people who were employed in other sectors. But they found it problematic that the projects had been defined as being concerned with health. One expressed it like this: 'The project was first and foremost a matter for the health services, they had little contact within the local authority.' Another stated that: 'When it comes to co-operating with the health services, I think it is wrong that the health sector should tell the other sectors what to do, it is a joint responsibility to develop the organisation.'

Similar strategies were chosen in the other community project. The health services defined the problems and also claimed they knew the solutions. The community projects very much 'led their own lives' within the health sector. There was what could be defined as a *medicalisation* of structural problems. This did not facilitate intersectoral co-operation. On the contrary, the other sectors found it alienating that structural problems were defined as health problems.

The environment projects

The situation was somewhat different in the environment projects. The municipalities were both urban cities. The environmental problems in both cities were defined as a major concern for the political authorities.

In both municipalities the project funding was used to employ a person within environmental health. Although they were employed within the health sector, their tasks made it necessary to co-operate with other sectors, especially with the environment advisor and the technical sector. The nature of co-operation was that experts met on equal terms.

In both municipalities the project workers took part in intersectoral co-operation. In one of them he was placed as a staff member with the Director for Health and Social Affairs. This gave him an opportunity to be a member of the municipal planning group for the environment. In the evaluation that was done by the project this was considered vital:

> Placing the project leader as a staff member with the Municipal Director turned out to be decisive for participating in a number of intersectoral projects. ... It was mostly planners, project

leaders and professionals who constituted a sort of lieutenant's rank and who took care of the intersectoral work.

At an early stage of the project, the health sector had a medicalisation strategy. This implied that they wanted to have a dominant position in environmental health care and they also wanted the health sector to play a dominant part in any intersectoral co-operation. The Medical Officer, who is the head of the health sector, put it like this in an interview: 'The Act of Municipal Health Services ... gives us a right and a duty to interfere with other people's business. Our task is to start processes and make things happen. This requires knowledge about social medicine.'

This attitude met resistance in the other sectors which did not want the health sector as a controller. The two following statements illustrate the reactions:

Sometimes it seems that the health sector wants as much as possible under its own hat. The question is when this will burst.

The health sector has got a problem within local authorities. They don't understand the difference between law and politics. They are only concerned about laws, but this is not the important thing for local authorities. A matter will also have to be made politically interesting to make local authorities prioritise it.

Eventually, the health sector changed its strategy and started to co-operate on equal terms. This, in turn, created a better climate for co-operation. Environmental health became a part of the environmental strategies in the municipality. This would, however, not be a special responsibility for the health sector, but for all sectors, and especially the political and administrative leadership.

This municipality was the only one in the present study where the project was actually continued after the Programme was over, that is, the municipality continued to fund the project. The other environment project was terminated, but there was a reorganisation where environment and environmental health became a central element in municipal plans and was also placed with the staff of the administrative municipality leadership.

The two community projects were both ended after the Programme was over. They had been quite isolated within the health sector and had little contact with other municipality sectors.

The projects were administered by the health services, but the strategies of co-operation with other sectors varied between the two types of projects. In the community projects the role of *controller* was chosen. This implied that even though the problems that were dealt with were vague, they were defined as medical problems.

As pointed out above, community work is at the borderline of public and civic sectors. The work is directed at the population and has no strict borders. It is, therefore, not easy to place these projects within the institutional framework of local authorities. In other words, it is not easy to continue a project when responsibilities are vague.

This was not the problem with the environmental care projects. On the contrary, they had a place within the framework of local authorities. The field was *institutionalised* as a public sector responsibility. They were compatible with the bureaucratic principles of public administration, and the projects therefore fitted more into the institutional framework of local authorities than was the case with the community projects. The differences between the two types are illustrated in Table 7.3.

Discussion and conclusion

In a decision perspective, the degree of change and the conflict/consensus of the policy are emphasised as factors influencing implementation. Especially at the state level, there were conflicts about

Table 7.3   Differences between community projects and environment health projects

Community projects	Environment projects
Borderline public/civic	Part of public sector
Not institutionalised	Institutionalised
Vague borders	Distinct borders
Population target group	Administration target group
Health sector as controller	Health sector as co-worker
Rural periphery	Urban central
Project theme not politicised	Project theme politicised

the National Programme. The Ministry of Health and Social Affairs and The National Board of Health had different and conflicting views on the Programme. The National Board wanted the health services to play a dominant role in health promotion. This would imply that the ideology of disease prevention would be dominant. This ideology emphasises the authority of experts and the role in co-operation would be that of the controller.

The Ministry wanted, however, an implementation of the WHO strategies. This would imply that the health services would have an equal, but not dominant, role in health promotion. The role of the health sector as co-worker is emphasised in this model.

The organisation at the central level seems to have influenced the outcome, especially the decision that the projects should be administered by the health services. The traditional role of the health services is the role of the experts advising the public. The organisation of the Programme gave an opportunity for the health sector to exercise the role of controller.

The process perspective allows an analysis of the process through the actions and ideologies of the actors who took part in the implementation process.

The different ideologies in the two project types may partly be explained by the different co-operation models that were chosen in the two projects. The community projects chose the role of controller, which indicated that the health service would be in charge of the projects and would define the problems. In the environment projects, however, the role of co-worker was adopted. This seemed more appropriate for facilitating intersectoral co-operation.

The theme of the projects also seems to play a significant role. The projects that were best implemented fitted well into the bureaucratic structure of local authorities. Their aim was to institutionalise environmental health as a public responsibility.

Community work, however, has a different character. Community participation and involvement are important, not to say dominant, strategies in the Ottawa Charter. The concept of empowerment, as it is understood by WHO, has its basis in community participation. This type of work has a different character from environmental health and does not fit into a bureaucratic administrative structure.

There seems to be two lessons to be learned from the Norwegian experience with the National Programme for Health Promotion. First, the health sector should not play a dominant part in these 'new' fields of health promotion. The model of disease prevention is not compatible with community work based on empowerment strategies. A bottom-up approach seems more in line with WHO's ideology than the top down model of disease prevention.

Second, it will be a challenge to integrate community health promotion into local authority structures. This represents, however, not only a challenge to health promotion workers, but also to central and local authorities. The traditional bureaucratic model of organisation does not seem to be compatible with the WHO ideologies of community action. A change of organisation and roles of civil servants who work within the local authority structure may be necessary if these ideologies are going to be implemented.

Notes

1 Local authorities in Denmark, Sweden and Great Britain have the opportunity to decide the level of local taxes. This is not the case in Norway, where tax limits are decided by central government.
2 The municipal sectors are usually health, social care, care for the elderly, school, culture and technical sector.
3 There are three income sources for local authorities: taxation, grants, and income sources like duties and fees. These are the same income sources as municipalities have in other European countries (Fimreite and Ryssevik 1998).
4 Until 1993 the name was the Directorate of Health.
5 The Ministry of Environment participated only in the initial phase.
6 The projects were dealing with health related environmental problems, such as indoor and outdoor pollution, noise, drinking water, etc.
7 In this respect I am referring to the Norwegian situation. In the late 1980s there was a National Programme called 'The Environment in the Municipalities'. The central government funded a post of Environment Advisor in all local authorities. The Programme was eventually turned into a permanent reform.

References

Baldersheim H. (1987) 'Kommunane – frå statstenar til stifinnar'. In: H.E. Næss *et al.* (eds) *Folkestyre i by og bygd*. Oslo: Universitetsforlaget.

Baldersheim H., Ståhlberg K. (eds) (1994) *Towards the Self-regulating Municipality*. Aldershot: Dartmouth.

Castongs C., Springett J. (1997) 'Towards a framework for the evaluation of health-related policies in cities'. *Evaluation* 3: 345–62.

Christensen T. (1994) *Politisk Styring og Faglig Uavhengighet. Reorganisering av den Sentrale Helseforvaltning*. Otta: Tano forlag.

Elmore R. (1979) 'Backward mapping: implementation research and policy decisions'. *Political Science Quarterly* 94: 601–16.

—— (1985) 'Forward and backward mapping: reversible logic in the analysis of public policy'. In K. Hanf, T. Toonen (eds) *Policy Implementation in Federal and Unitary Systems*. Dordrecht: Martinus Nijhof Publishers.

Fimreite A., Ryssevik J. (eds) (1998) *Kommunal Monitor.* Norsk Samfunnsvitenskapelig datatjeneste. Bergen.

Helsedirektoratet (1989) *Samlet Plan for Utviklingsprosjekter Innen det Sykdomsforebyggende og Helsefremmende Arbeid.*

Hjern B. (1982) 'Implementation research – the link gone missing'. *Journal of Public Policy* 2: 301–8.

Hjern B., Hull C. (1982) 'Implementation research as empirical constitutionalism'. *European Journal of Political Research* 10: 105–15.

Hjern B., Porter D. (1981) 'Implementation structures: a new unit of administrative analysis'. *Organization Studies* 2/3: S211–27.

Huberman M., Miles M. (1994) 'Data management and analysis methods'. In N. Denzin, Y. Lincoln (eds) *Handbook of Qualitative Research.* London: Sage.

Jensen J. (1983) *Sygdomsbegreber i Praxis.* København: Munkgsgaard forlag.

Kjellberg F. (1991) 'Kommunalt selvstyre og nasjonal styring. Mot nye roller for kommunene?' *Norsk Statsvitenskapelig Tidsskrift* 7: 45–63.

Kjellberg F., Reitan M. (1995) *Studiet av Offentlig Politikk – en Innføring.* Otta: Tano forlag.

Kommunenøkkelen 1996.

Mazmanian D., Sabatier P. (1981) *Effective Policy Implementation.* Lexington, Massachusetts: D.C. Heath and Company.

Milward B. (1982) 'Interorganizational policy systems and research on public organizations'. *Administration and Society* 13: S457–78.

Nordby T. (1987) 'Profesjokratiets periode innen norsk helsevesen – institusjoner, politikk og konfliktemner'. *Historisk Tidsskrift* 3.

Pawson R., Tilley N. (1997) *Realistic Evaluation.* London: Sage.

Pressmann J., Wildavsky A. (1973) *Implementation.* Berkeley: University of California Press.

Rimpelä M. (1984) *Preventive Medicine vs. Health Promotion. An Overview of Historical Trends.* Department of Public Health, University of Helsinki.

Rouban L. (1993) 'Public administration and political change'. *International Political Science Review* 14: 315–318

Sabatier P. (1986) 'Top down and bottom up approaches to implementation research. A critical analysis and suggested synthesis'. *Journal of Public Policy* 6: 21–48.

Stortingsmelding nr. 41 (1987–88) *Helsepolitikken mot år 2000.*

Stortingsmelding nr. 6 (1989–9) *Røynsler med Lova om Helsetenesta i Kommunane.*

Stortingsmelding nr. 37 (1992–93) *Utfordringer i Helsefremmende og Forebyggende Arbeid.*

van Meter D., van Horn C. (1975) 'The policy implementation process. A conceptual framework'. *Administration and Society* 6: 4.

Winter S. (1990) 'Integrating implementation research'. In: D.J. Palumbo and D.J. Calista (eds) *Implementation and the Policy Process. Opening up the Black Box*. New York: Greenwood Press.

Chapter 8

Does health economics do health promotion justice?

Janine Hale

Introduction

Economics exist because choices have to be made; scarcity is one of the key concepts in economics. The nature of the choices differs according to the level at which decisions are made. As individuals we have limited time and money and therefore have to make choices about how we spend our limited incomes and how we allocate our limited time to various activities. At a collective level choices have to be made about how scarce resources should be employed to achieve varieties of different outputs. Economic principles can be used to explain and predict decisions at the individual level and to aid decision-making at the organisational level.

It is becoming increasingly accepted that resources for health care are scarce and therefore choices in the health care sector have to be made. One criterion upon which these choices can be based is efficiency, i.e. maximising the benefit to any resource expenditure, or minimising the cost of any achieved benefit. In economics, cost refers to the principle that when a choice is made to use resources in one way, those resources can no longer be used in another way. The benefit that could be achieved by using them in an alternative programme is therefore foregone. The (opportunity) cost is the foregone benefit from the next best alternative.

In view of the above, it is common for interventions/health care technologies to be subject to economic evaluation prior to implementation on a wide scale. Health promotion activities make claims on resources that could be put to alternative uses. It is important, therefore, that these activities are subjected to the same evaluation requirements as other health care methodologies in order to maximise the health gains from available resources. There are, however, fewer evaluations of health promotion activities than other health care programmes (Buck *et al.* 1996), and it is often stated that applying the standard economic appraisal techniques to health promotion discriminates against it (Barry and De Friese 1990). One of the aims of this chapter is to outline the role health economics can play in helping to evaluate health promotion programmes and to illustrate the difficulties encountered when applying the standard economic evaluation techniques, such as discounting, identification and measurement of benefits etc.

Whilst health economics clearly has an important role to play in the evaluation of health promotion programmes, that is not the only level at which decisions are made. Individuals are also faced with having to make choices. The role of health economics at this level has been neglected even further. Whilst there are examples in the literature of economic theories of the demand for health (Grossman 1972, Cropper 1977, Muurinen 1982, Wagstaff 1986, Dardanoni and Wagstaff 1987), these have been little used within health promotion to help explain individuals' decisions regarding health promoting behaviour.

The second aim of this chapter is to illustrate how the concepts and principles of economics can contribute to explaining individuals' choices regarding health affecting behaviour using one model (the 'Utility Model of Preventive Behaviour' (Cohen 1984), as an example.

Health economics as an aid to evaluation

Economic appraisal is a set of methods for examining alternative courses of action with a view to helping make a choice. It is meant as an aid to decision-making, not a replacement for it. The criterion most often used is economic efficiency, which concerns the relationship between resource inputs and outputs.

There are four levels of economic appraisal; cost benefit analysis is the broadest, and cost minimisation analysis the narrowest. As we move between the methods, the data requirements change, as does the information provided by the evaluation and the implications for health promotion.

Cost benefit analysis

Cost benefit analysis expresses all gains and sacrifices in common units (usually money) allowing a judgement to be made as to whether, or to what extent, an objective should be pursued. At this level of analysis the objective can be questioned.

The definition of costs and benefits is very wide; the costs of the programme are all the resources which have alternative uses, i.e. where opportunity costs are incurred, and not just money spent, and benefits are all that results that is of value. In the first instance, the chosen perspective is that of society, where all costs are accounted for regardless of who bears them and all benefits are included regardless of to whom they accrue. The concern is whether the community as a whole bears a cost, not who pays for it, and similarly, whether the community as a whole benefits.

Full cost benefit analyses are not often undertaken due to the large data requirements, and the difficulty of placing a monetary value on some of the benefits. There are, however, examples in the literature of partial analyses, for example, of smoking cessation in pregnancy (Ershoff *et al.* 1990, Marks *et al.* 1990, Windsor *et al.* 1993), where the resource savings from fewer low birth-weight babies are so great that they outweigh the costs of the smoking cessation programme. In such cases, there is no need to value the health effects to either mother or child from quitting.

In most instances, economists define the costs and benefits to a community as the sums of the costs and benefits accruing to all individuals in that community. With the increasing emphasis on community development and social capital, however, this may not be the most appropriate view of community to use. Indeed there needs to be development in the whole area of community evaluation (Shiell and Hawe 1996).

Defining the objective

There is a common misunderstanding among health promotion specialists and others that economics is about money. This results in the idea that economists assume that the objective of health promotion is (or should be) to save money (Pelletier 1991, Lynch and Vickery 1993), as the following, not untypical, quote shows.

While there is considerable scope for investment of resources in better economic analyses, it is important to bear in mind that the purpose of health education, and health promotion generally, is not simply to save money.

(Reid 1996)

Economics is about the relationship between resource inputs and outputs, with costs being only one side of the equation. It is not the economist's role to determine the objective of a given programme. The objective needs to be defined before the most appropriate outcome measure can be identified. The broader the objective, the broader will be the range of benefits. Economic evaluation techniques need to be able to recognise that there may be multiple objectives in health promotion, with different outcome measures being appropriate at different levels (Nutbeam 1998).

The benefits of health promotion

For the purposes of economic evaluation a benefit is defined as anything that results that is of value (and strictly, that individuals would be willing to pay for) (Drummond 1980).

There are two main difficulties that arise when considering the benefits of health promotion programmes. The first is identification. One view of health promotion is that a successful health promotion programme results in the prevention of ill health. However, there is no way of identifying for certain what amount would have arisen in the absence of the programme under consideration. The attribution of the outcomes to the intervention is complicated in health promotion programmes by the long time delay between implementation of the programme and any reduction in morbidity or mortality. In the case of clinical interventions, attribution is less of a problem, both because there is a shorter time between intervention and effect, and because of the ability to use randomised control trials to observe the effect. It is now becoming well recognised that this evaluation framework is not appropriate for the majority of health promotion programmes (WHO 1998).

There is also the possibility of wider benefits than those originally identified in the evaluation. For example, a health promotion programme aimed at reducing heart disease may have additional benefits in its effects on the risks for other illnesses, which may be overlooked in the evaluation. The possibility of social diffusion, where one person changing their behaviour as a result of a health promotion campaign may result in others around them also changing their behaviour, also needs to be considered. For example, Rosen (1989) estimated the impact of social diffusion on smoking to be 20 per cent, which implies that for every ten people who stop smoking there will be another two who also stop, or do not start.

A further example of a potentially missed benefit is provided by the possibility of a 'lifestyle effect' of regular exercise, where an individual who undertakes regular exercise also changes other aspects of their lifestyle, making them more healthy too (Wester-Wedman 1988). There are also externalities or interpersonal external effects (Sugden and Williams 1978). These occur when an individual gains a benefit from the knowledge that others have received the health promotion programme, even if that individual does not receive the programme themselves.

The second difficulty is with measurement. Since cost benefit analysis should in principle include all costs and benefits, then *short term* benefits from health promotion, such as increased energy resulting from an increase in exercise, or greater self-esteem due to weight loss ought to be included, in addition to benefits in terms of final health outcomes which are anticipated.

One difficulty with cost benefit analysis is that it expresses all costs and benefits in the same units, i.e. a value needs to be placed on these benefits in money terms. There are techniques available to help with this, such as willingness to pay (Berwick and Weinstein 1985, Donaldson 1990), where an individual is asked to state the maximum amount they would be willing to pay to receive a certain benefit. This has the added advantage of identifying which of the hypothesised benefits are in fact perceived as such by those receiving them. For example, it may be hypothesised that giving individuals information is a benefit even if it does not lead to a change in behaviour, whereas the individuals themselves may not be willing to pay a positive price for the information they have received. In some instances individuals could feel worse off after having received the information due to increased anxiety.

Cost effectiveness analysis

Cost effectiveness analysis requires fewer data than cost benefit analysis, and is much easier to carry out. As such, examples can be found more easily in the literature (for example, see Baxter *et al.* 1997, Ratcliffe *et al.* 1997, Field *et al.* 1995, Altman *et al.* 1987,

Phillips 1997), although they are still relatively uncommon in the area of health promotion (Buck *et al.* 1996).

Cost effectiveness analysis takes a narrower perspective, focusing on the best way of meeting a stated objective given that some means of pursuing it is going ahead. The objective of the programme is not being, and cannot be, questioned by a cost effectiveness analysis. The most cost effective alternative is that which achieves a given benefit at lowest cost, or gives the greatest benefit for a given expenditure, but here benefits are expressed in terms of narrowly specified units of effectiveness only. The question being considered now is one of technical efficiency: given that a programme is going ahead, which is the best way of doing it? Only programmes with the same objective and producing the same unit of effectiveness can be compared using this technique. As with benefits in cost benefit analysis, the chosen output measure must be perceived in terms of the objective. For example, if the objective is to encourage people to quit smoking, then the number of quitters is a valid measure of output. Resource savings from fewer smoking related diseases, or health benefits of extending life, need not be considered in cost effectiveness analysis. The extent to which single output appraisals are appropriate for health promotion programmes which may have multiple objectives needs to be carefully considered and the results of cost effectiveness analyses of such programmes can be potentially very misleading.

Cost utility analysis

The third technique of economic appraisal is cost utility analysis, which is a form of cost effectiveness analysis where benefits are measured in terms of a utility measure such as the quality adjusted life year (QALY). Using a measure such as the QALY assumes that all programmes have the same ultimate objective – to maximise health gain. Some authors argue that these are inappropriate for use in evaluating health promotion programmes (Cribb and Haycox 1989, Jan and Mooney 1997). There is certainly difficulty using these in health promotion, since the starting point here is an essentially healthy population. QALY measures are unlikely to pick up many of the short-term changes which result from a health promotion campaign, such as the greater self-esteem due to weight loss or the increase in energy from undertaking an exercise programme. When using these measures in programmes of treatment and cure there is the advantage that these programmes often have a condition specific measure that can be used alongside the generic QALYs – something that health promotion does not.

Cost utility analysis allows comparisons across different programmes, so providing more information than a standard cost effectiveness analysis, but not having all the difficulties of a full cost benefit analysis. This technique has the advantage that there is no need to put a monetary value on the outcome (QALY), but the disadvantage that many of the benefits that may result are still being ignored. To the extent that cost effectiveness analysis may be inappropriate for health promotion, the same can also be said of cost utility analysis. Whilst using a QALY measure has the advantage that a broader objective can be pursued than in many cost effectiveness analyses, this is outweighed by the current difficulty of using these measures in this area.

Cost minimisation analysis

The final form of economic appraisal is cost minimisation analysis – this is performed when the outcomes of two interventions cannot differ. However, it is seldom the case that it is known that the outcomes cannot differ and so cost minimisation analyses are rare, and virtually non-existent in the case of health promotion.

One overall message that is emerging is that careful consideration needs to be given in economic appraisal to the choice of final outcome measure so that important outputs from health promotion activity are not ignored. The wider the outcome measure that can be used, the greater the range of benefits that can be included in the appraisal.

Of all the difficulties mentioned so far, only one is a result of the economics – that is the need to place a value on the benefits. The problems of determining the objective and identifying and measuring benefits are problems of evaluation *per se* and need to be resolved even if economists do not get involved. There is, however, one other issue that is part of economic evaluation that is the cause of much contention and confusion (and resentment) among health promotion specialists (West 1996), namely the issue of discounting.

Differential timing of costs and benefits

One problem that needs to be addressed in economic evaluation, which is particularly relevant for health promotion, is the fact that costs and benefits rarely occur at the same point in time. In economics it is widely recognised that people have preferences over the timing of costs and benefits, preferring benefits now and costs later (Drummond 1980). In recognition of these time preferences, an adjustment needs to be made so that like is compared with like. This adjustment is called 'discounting'. The process of discounting future costs and benefits to their present values is often criticised, and it is often argued that this discriminates against health promotion' (West 1996).

In conventional economic appraisal in the UK future benefits and costs are normally discounted at a rate recommended by the Treasury, currently 6 per cent. While there is little disagreement with this in the case of monetary benefits and costs, there remains much controversy over whether future intangible health benefits yielded by programmes in health care should be discounted at some different rate, if at all. Some economists have argued for a zero or near zero rate for health benefits (Parsonage and Neuberger 1992), while others have defended the use of a common rate for health and wealth (Williams 1981, Keeler and Cretin 1983) and most things in between. It cannot be disputed that if a positive discount rate is used, this gives greater weight to costs and benefits occurring earlier (Sugden and Williams 1978). High discount rates will therefore tend to work against those alternatives with costs occurring today and benefits occurring relatively late, as is often the case with health promotion (this point may be of particular relevance if health promotion is being compared with clinical interventions).

One suggested way to resolve this problem is to discount in the usual way, but to use a range of values including zero to assess what effect this has on the result (Tolley 1993). Whilst this presents both sides of the argument, it contributes little to solving the debate – the final decision as to which result to use still needs to be made – and the implications of different rates being used still exist.

Using a zero rate implicitly assumes that society has no preference between present and future benefits. Commissioners certainly have preferences for present benefits imposed on them by the nature of their budgets.

Tolley (1993) also suggests that the problem of the differential timing of costs and benefits could be overcome by concentrating on the short-term health benefits of health promotion. This is entirely in keeping with the economic way of thinking which defines a benefit as anything that results that is of value. This does, however, bring us back to the difficulties of identification and measurement. An outcome measure which picks up all aspects of the benefits from health promotion activity, both long term and short term, is clearly needed. The effect of discounting on a stream of benefits starting now and continuing into the future is much less pronounced than the effect on a benefit occurring ten or twenty years from now. This would have the added advantage of partly overcoming the short-term view imposed on commissioners by their budgets, demonstrating the benefits that are being gained now.

The issue of discounting is one that still attracts much debate in health economics. There is increasing evidence to suggest that the constant discounting model most frequently used is not the most appropriate, and models of decreasing timing aversion should be considered instead (Cairns and Van der Pol 1997), i.e. less importance is placed on a one-year difference between years twenty and twenty-one than a one-year difference between years five and six. Alternative discounting models are beginning to be investigated (ibid. 1997) and need in particular to be further investigated in the area of health promotion.

Decision-making at the individual level

Health economics has an important role to play in the evaluation of health promotion programmes, but that is not the only level at which decisions are made. As indicated earlier, individuals are also faced with having to make choices. Economics can contribute to explaining individuals' choices regarding health affecting behaviour. This will be illustrated using one model as an example.

Economics is a behavioural science and can be used to explain how on the basis of individual preferences, individuals make decisions about which goods and services to consume subject to their personal income constraint. While there are several psycho-social theories about health promoting behaviour (Becker 1974, Becker and Maiman 1975, Becker et al. 1977), there has been little effort to use economics to explain why individuals demand (or do not demand) things that are good or bad for them (i.e. which affect their risks of future ill health or injury). Cohen and Mooney (1984) have defined preventive and hazardous goods as goods (and services) whose consumption alters the risk of future illness or injury. Unlike most goods, however, the consumption of prevention and hazard goods results in two types of utility (satisfaction): utility-in-antici-pation, from the increased peace of mind resulting from the consumption of prevention goods; and utility-in-use, the utility obtained directly from consuming both prevention and hazard goods.

These ideas were further developed by Cohen (1984) into the 'Utility Model of Preventive Behaviour'. Cohen argued that many goods which affect the risks of future ill-health are consumed for reasons that are not preventive at all, but which are nevertheless prevention goods by definition. Examples could include wholemeal bread or exercise, both of which may be consumed for reasons of utility-in-use (i.e. they yield pleasure) independent of any effect they may have on future risk. It was suggested that the non-preventive reasons for undertaking preventive behaviour may have an import-ant role to play in explaining, predicting and trying to change these behaviours.

To date, this model remains untested. Nevertheless, it still provides a useful example of how economics can be used to explore individual health affecting behaviour. Health affecting behaviour, which is expressed in terms of the demand for prevention goods and hazard goods, is different from the demand for all other goods and services because of 'utility-in-anticipation' which only occurs in the case of these goods. Cohen (1984) points out that utility-in-antici-pation is a stream of utility starting *immediately* after the prevention takes place, and continuing until the time when the outcome was expected. Total utility is the sum of the utility-in-anticipation and the utility-in-use, both of which can be positive, zero or negative. As with all other goods and services, economic theory would suggest that the prevention good will be consumed if the total utility is greater than the cost.

Since total utility is made up of utility-in-use and utility-in-anticipation, there are essentially three elements that can be targeted if the objective is to change behaviour: utility-in-anticipation, utility-in-use and cost (Cohen 1984).

A health promotion programme whose aim is to change behaviour can adopt either of two approaches depending on the relative weights of each type of utility – and this will vary between different groups in society. For example, young people who tend to have high time preference rates are less likely to be influenced by a programme highlighting the health benefits of avoiding cancer in fifty years time (and the stream of utility in anticipation to be gained during that period) than they are by attempting to reduce the utility-in-use they get by smoking (e.g. by emphasising that smoking annoys other people and causes bad breath).

It is the relative amounts of utility-in-use and utility-in-anticipation that are important in the context of prevention goods. If this can be determined, it becomes easier to design the programme that is likely to have the greatest impact.

Finally, since the consumption decision is based on a weighing up of the utility and cost, the cost side of the equation can be manipulated by subsidising the cost of prevention goods and taxing hazard goods.

Discussion

In summary, economics has an important role to play in health promotion on two levels. The first and most often considered is as an aid to evaluation. There are difficulties applying the standard and accepted techniques, especially in terms of the specification of an objective and the identification and measurement of the benefits. These difficulties are not unique to the economic evaluation, but health economists need to develop a better understanding of health promotion and recognise that there may be more than one objective and hence different levels of outcome to use. Further work needs to be done on using techniques to value the benefits to facilitate cost benefit analyses, rather than focusing on a single restricted unit of effectiveness. The second role is that of a behavioural science, helping to explain from an economic perspective how individuals decide to undertake health affecting behaviour. The model used as an example illustrates how economics can explain individual behaviour, which in turn can be used to tailor health promotion programmes to particular target groups in society.

So, does health economics do health promotion justice? The concentration on a single long-term unit of effectiveness in cost-effectiveness analysis has probably not done health promotion justice. This is not, however, entirely the fault of the health economist. Specification of the objective of health promotion is not the health economist's role. If appraisals that have been carried out have concentrated on a single objective and a single (inappropriate) output measure, it is the responsibility of the health promotion specialists to correct this misunderstanding.

To overcome these difficulties and for health promotion to

benefit from what economics has to offer, collaboration between health economists and health promotion specialists would seem to be essential. It will take involvement and input from health promotion specialists and health economists to find the best methods of adapting the standard techniques to suit health promotion better. Time and energy need to be devoted to developing an outcome measure similar to the QALY for health promotion which captures the full range of benefits available from a health promotion programme so that they can be included in cost utility analyses. Consideration should also be given to the possibility of doing more and more comprehensive cost benefit analyses instead of cost effectiveness analyses, which involves identifying, measuring and valuing all costs and benefits resulting from a health promotion programme. These suggestions are not a quick fix to the difficulties posed by applying the standard economic appraisal techniques to health promotion programmes. If it is felt that the way health economics has been used to date has not done health promotion justice then collaboration between the two disciplines must be the only way forward.

Acknowledgement

My thanks go to David Cohen, at the University of Glamorgan, and Chris Tudor-Smith and Chris Roberts, at Health Promotion Wales, for comments on earlier drafts of this work. Any errors are solely those of the author.

References

Altman D.G., Flora J.A., Fortmann S.P., Farquhar J.W. (1987) 'The cost-effectiveness of three smoking cessation programs'. *American Journal of Public Health* 77: 162–5.

Barry P., De Friese G. (1990) 'Cost-benefit and cost-effectiveness analysis for health promotion programs'. *American Journal of Health Promotion* 4: 448–52.

Baxter T., Milner P., Wilson K., Leaf M., Nicholl J., Freeman J., Cooper N. (1997) 'A cost effective community based heart health promotion project in England: prospective comparative study'. *BMJ* 315: 582–5.

Becker M.H. (ed.) (1974) 'The health belief model and personal health behaviour'. *Health Education Monograph* 2.

Becker M.H., Maiman L.A. (1975) 'Sociobehavioural determinants of compliance with health and medical recommendations'. *Medical Care* 13: 10–24.

Becker M.H., Haefner D.P., Kasl S.V., Kirscht J.P., Maiman L.A., Rosenstock I.M. (1977) 'Selected psychological models and correlates of individual health related behaviour'. *Medical Care* 15: S27–S46.

Berwick D.M., Weinstein M.C. (1985) 'What do patients value? Willingness to pay for ultrasound in pregnancy'. *Medical Care* 23: 881–93.

Buck D., Godfrey C., Killoran A., Tolley K. (1996) 'Reducing the burden of coronary heart disease: health promotion, its effectiveness and cost'. *Health Education Research* 11: 487–99.

Cairns J., Van Der Pol M. (1997) 'Saving future lives. A comparison of three discounting models'. *Health Economics* 6: 341–50.

Cohen D.R. (1984) 'Utility model of preventive behaviour'. *Journal of Epidemiology and Community Health* 38: 61–5.

Cohen D.R., Mooney G.H. (1984) 'Prevention goods and hazard goods: a taxonomy'. *Scottish Journal of Political Economy* 31: 92–9.

Cribb A., Haycox A. (1989) 'Economic analysis in the evaluation of health promotion'. *Community Medicine* 11: 299–305.

Cropper M.L. (1977) 'Health, investment in health and occupational choice'. *Journal of Political Economy* 85: 1,273–95.

Dardanoni V., Wagstaff A. (1987) 'Uncertainty, inequalities in health and the demand for health'. *Journal of Health Economics* 6: 283–90.

Donaldson C. (1990) 'Willingness to pay for publicly-provided goods. A possible measure of benefit?' *Journal of Health Economics* 9: 103–18.

Drummond M.F. (1980) *Principles of Economic Appraisal in Health Care*. Oxford: Oxford University Press.

Ershoff D.H., Quinn V.P., Dolan Mullen P., Lairson D.R. (1990) 'Pregnancy and medical cost outcomes of a self-help prenatal smoking cessation program in a HMO'. *Public Health Reports* 105: 340–7.

Field K., Thorogood M., Silagy C., Normand C., O'Neill C., Muir J. (1995) 'Strategies for reducing coronary risk factors in primary care: which is most cost-effective?' *BMJ* 310: 1,109–12.

Grossman M. (1972) 'On the concept of health capital and the demand for health'. *Journal of Political Economy* 80: 223–55.

Jakarta Declaration on Leading Health Promotion into the 21st Century (1997) *Health Promotion International* 12: 261–4.

Jan S., Mooney G. (1997) 'The outcomes of health promotion: are QALYs enough?' *Health Promotion Journal of Australia* 7: 88–90.

Keeler E.B., Cretin S. (1983) 'Discounting of life-saving and other non-monetary effects'. *Management Science* 29: 300–6.

Lynch W.P., Vickery D.M. (1993) 'The potential impact of health promotion on health care utilisation: an introduction to demand management'. *American Journal of Health Promotion* 8: 87–92.

Marks J.S., Kaplan J.P., Hogue C.J-R., Dalmat M.E. (1990) 'A cost-benefit/cost-effectiveness analysis of smoking cessation for pregnant women'. *American Journal of Preventive Medicine* 6: 282–9.

Muurinen J.M. (1982) 'Demand for health: a generalised Grossman model'. *Journal of Health Economics* 1: 5–28.

Nutbeam D. (1998) 'Evaluating health promotion – progress, problems and solutions'. *Health Promotion International* 13: 27–44.

Parsonage M., Neuberger H. (1992) 'Discounting and health benefits'. *Health Economics* 1: 71–9.

Pelletier K.R. (1991) 'A review and analysis of the health and cost-effective outcome studies of comprehensive health promotion and disease prevention programs'. *American Journal of Health Promotion* 5: 311–15.

Phillips C. (1997) *Economic Evaluation and Health Promotion.* Aldershot: Avebury.

Ratcliffe J., Cairns J., Platt S. (1997) 'Cost effectiveness of a mass media-led anti-smoking campaign in Scotland'. *Tobacco Control* 6: 104–10.

Reid D. (1996) 'How effective is health education via mass communications?' *Health Education Journal* 55: 332–44.

Rosen M. (1989) 'On randomised controlled trials and lifestyle intervention'. *International Journal of Epidemiology* 18: 993–4.

Shiell A., Hawe P. (1996) 'Health promotion community development and the tyranny of individualism'. *Health Economics* 5: 241–7.

Sugden R., Williams A. (1978) *The Principles of Practical Cost-Benefit Analysis.* Oxford: Oxford University Press.

Tolley K. (1993) *Health Promotion: How to Measure Cost-Effectiveness.* London: Health Education Authority.

Wagstaff A. (1986) 'The demand for health. Some new empirical evidence'. *Journal of Health Economics* 5: 195–233.

West R. (1996) 'Discounting the future: influence of the economic model'. *Journal of Epidemiology and Community Health* 50: 239–44.

Wester-Wedman A. (1988) 'The elusive jogger. A study of the process of establishing regular physical exercising habits'. In: M. Rosen and L. Lindholm (eds) 'The neglected effects of lifestyle interventions in cost-effectiveness analysis'. *Health Promotion International* 1992 7(3): 163–9.

Williams A. (1981) 'Welfare economics and health status measurement'. In: J. van der Gaag, M. Perlman (eds) *Health, Economics and Health Economics.* North Holland.

World Health Organization (WHO) European Working Group on Health Promotion Evaluation (1998) *Health Promotion Evaluation: Recommendations to Policymakers.*

Windsor R.A., Lowe J.B., Perkins L.L., Smith-Yoder D., Artz L., Crawford M., Amburgy J., Boyd Jr. N.R. (1993) 'Health education for pregnant smokers: its behavioural impact and cost benefit'. *American Journal of Public Health* 83: 201–6.

Part III

Good practice

Based on previous discussion we can begin to identify certain criteria by which good practice can be judged. In this final part of the book, findings from five studies are presented.

In Chapter 9 Marcelo Ramella and Jennifer Attride-Stirling describe an innovative project on young people's sexual health promotion in Peru. On the basis of preliminary findings, the authors explore the effectiveness of implementing a community-based, action research approach, its theoretical foundations and methodological provisions. Health in general, and sexual health in particular, are understood as resources for living, indivisible from other community resources, for example, economic or emotional. The actualisation of sexual health promotion takes place via adolescent networks steered by the youths themselves, organised in 'gendered spaces', created and developed through an open, multi-layered process encompassing various social dimensions. Key to the functioning of these spaces are, first, that they are owned by the youth, and, second, that their contents and boundaries are subjected to continual negotiation within the community. It is proposed that gendered spaces provide an effective medium for the promotion of sexual health in a culturally sensitive fashion. Experiences taking place in the adolescent networks are recorded and interpreted by the youth with the aid of multimedia technologies, providing the raw data for research. The authors suggest that a systematised application of this technology in the field of sexual health promotion research constitutes a fertile methodology for enhancing academic and practitioner understanding of youth sexual health practices, concerns and needs.

The study by Vivien Swanson and Kevin Power (Chapter 10) aimed to predict determinants of infant feeding behaviour using a theoretically based social cognition approach. The relationship between feeding beliefs, normative values, behavioural control, feeding intention and infant feeding behaviour was assessed for new mothers within forty-eight hours of delivery in hospitals in rural and urban settings in Scotland. Partners' beliefs and attitudes were also measured. A corresponding pilot study in Greece enabled cross-cultural comparisons of model components. The decision to breast or bottlefeed was made before conception for most mothers in the Scottish and Greek samples. For the Scottish sample, beliefs about infant feeding were the strongest predictor of breast-feeding in hospital. Partners' beliefs, social norms and previous breast-feeding were, however, also significant predictors. Comparisons of breast and bottlefeeders in Scotland revealed significant differences in feeding beliefs, partners' beliefs, social norms and behavioural control over the decision to breast or bottlefeed. The authors conclude that a structured theoretical social cognition approach is useful in predicting infant feeding behaviour and identifying cross-cultural differences in beliefs, social norms and control over the feeding decision. Early, school-based educational intervention may be most effective in promoting positive beliefs about breast-feeding.

A recent systematic review of health promotion interventions among gay men judged only five studies, all conducted in the USA, to be methodologically sound. Two of these studies successfully used peer educators in gay bars to endorse HIV risk reduction among other gay men. In response to the recommendation of the review, that interventions using peer educators should be explored further in well-designed evaluations in the UK, an appropriate intervention has been developed and is described in Chapter 11 by Jonathan Elford, Lorraine Sherr and Graham Bolding. The 4 gym project is targeted at gay men attending one of four gyms (all with a large gay membership) in central London. The project recruited peer educators from people who use the gym regularly. After attending a training course they undertake to talk to 20–25 gay men at their gym over the subsequent four- to five-month period about HIV prevention, focusing on safer sex and steroid use (particularly injecting and needle sharing). The intervention is being evaluated by means of a controlled trial which has three 6-month phases. All men attending the gyms will be asked at regular intervals (baseline, 6-, 12- and 18-month follow-up) to complete a questionnaire on sexual risk behaviour and steroid use. Information collected from these questionnaires will indicate whether there has been any change in sexual or injecting risk behaviour following the intervention. If found to be effective, peer-led HIV prevention programmes could be introduced into other venues such as bars and clubs. The chapter details the methodology that underpins the investigation, presents process-related material concerning the intervention and the evaluation and describes preliminary baseline findings.

Chapter 12 by Cicely Kerr, Jenny Maslin, Jim Orford, Sue Dalton, Maria Ferrins-Brown and Elizabeth Hartney reports the process and findings of a three-stage, grounded theory analysis of alcohol health education conducted as part of the Birmingham Untreated Heavy Drinkers Project. Quantitative and qualitative data were gathered from a community sample of 500 male and female regular drinkers via a confidential interview. The exploration of participants' views of alcohol-focused health education messages was one of several areas contained within the interview. Data from a subsample of 62 participants were analysed for emerging themes, and a model of how these individuals have internalised and acted on alcohol health messages was formulated. The model reveals that, despite awareness of the health risks of excessive drinking, moderation of consumption is barred by low perception of severity of health risks, low deterrent effect of health risks, valued benefits of current drinking and low perceived control over drinking, although harm reduction behaviours are being practised. The model and its implications for health education messages is discussed with reference to models of health behaviour and recent alcohol education messages.

In the final chapter of the book, Anne MacFarlane and Cecily Kelleher report the findings of a study which examines previous and current health beliefs, health behaviours and pluralistic responses to illness among older people in Ireland. The stated purpose of the study is to increase knowledge and understanding of motivating factors underlying both professional and non-professional responses to illness. Fifty-one older people (aged 69–72 years), recruited from a representative national survey, participated in a postal and interview study. Perceived generational differences in health behaviour were discussed by participants in relation to diet, activity and psychosocial factors. Contemporary sedentary lifestyles were contrasted with accounts of health enhancing lifestyles of participants' childhood years. The socio-cultural context of lifestyles was noted within these data. Changing trends in medical practices were discussed in terms of presenting conditions, treatment availability and utilisation patterns in terms of reported knowledge and use. Critical attitudes about contemporary health service utilisation by the current generation were expressed. Views about appropriate utilisation reflected ideas about necessity as dictated by symptom severity. A decline in traditional Irish folk medicine and an increased reliance on biomedicine was evident among participants and explained in terms of treatment availability but, also, socio-cultural norms surrounding utilisation of professional and non-professional medical systems. These findings are discussed in relation to the practice and theory of health promotion in terms of health promotion initiatives for older people and the limits of existing socio-psychological models and constructs.

Chapter 9

The creation of gendered spaces as a medium for sexual health promotion among young people in Peru

Marcelo Ramella and
Jennifer Attride-Stirling

Introduction

Sexual health promotion is to a large and crucial extent about facilitating shared decisions; adolescent sexual health promotion constitutes a paradigmatic case. In working with adolescents the issue of sexual health promotion acquires extra layers of complexity, particularly as much of the scientific literature on the topic has often failed to capture the reality of the adolescents, who rarely have the opportunity to elaborate this reality themselves.[1] Moreover, adolescent sexual health promotion involves an array of unsettled and delicate issues ranging from age and gender to various taboos that touch conflicting points lying at the intersection of the socio-cultural, the medical and the legal spheres (Griffin 1993).

Initiatives oriented to promoting sexual health among adolescents have traditionally tended to focus on the content of the decisions at stake, neglecting both their shared nature as well as innumerable aspects that facilitate or hinder the decision-making process. As a result there is a worrying record of failure in the short but prolific history of adolescent sexual health promotion (UNFPA 1997, Senderowitz 1995, Milburn 1996, Atkin *et al.* 1996). Furthermore, failed interventions may, in addition to or instead of solving the problems identified, produce side effects with long lasting negative impact on the adolescents and the communities.

Giving centrality to local cultures, to adolescent participation and to the shared and facilitation aspects of decision processes, the chapter attempts to provide a social psychological approach to the issue of sexual health promotion among adolescents. Focusing on a project that is being carried out in severely deprived areas of Peru, we propose the concept of the gendered space as an effective medium for the promotion of adolescent sexual health. The gendered space is conceptualised as a community-grounded social sphere where interaction, exchange and dialogue between young women and men are facilitated. This central notion is based on the contention that reflexivity and change are best enacted via open communication among stakeholders (Freire 1972, Habermas 1996, Foucault 1987), and adolescent sexual health promotion needs fundamentally to take this into account.

The notion of gendered space provides a promising tool for the promotion of sexual health among adolescents. It combines in an innovative fashion a fundamentally social conceptualisation of health promotion, with a challenging approach to adolescent participation. Indeed, in the gendered space the promotion of sexual health is indivisible from the everyday social life of the community. Local resources, material as much as normative and emotional, become the lifeblood of the health promotion process, constantly flowing in and out of the gendered space. The adolescents, in turn, become the main agents in this process of health promotion as it is they who shape agendas, take decisions and enact change.

This chapter outlines the theoretical basis underpinning the approach, discusses preliminary findings corresponding to the first two years of implementation of the project, and sketches further steps to be carried out in the future. It proposes some ideas that might be of use for practitioners, and of interest to researchers in the field of adolescent sexual health promotion. Although the bulk of the chapter relies on evidence from communities located in environments which suffer from sharp imbalances in the distribution of resources – wealth as much as health – many of the ideas and concepts discussed can well apply to communities and circumstances elsewhere.

What are gendered spaces?

Gendered spaces have been conceived as change-enabling social spheres, rooted in the community, where dialogue, negotiation and active collaboration between young men and women are encouraged and facilitated. Of course, the fact that there are men and women involved is not the sole reason for the 'gendered' quality of this social space, as the term has been employed to call attention to the multitude of intertwined significations inhabiting the lives of these women and men: friend, carer, worker, nurturer, provider, partner, etc. (Collier 1995). This space aims to host, as much as to provoke, collective debate and collective action by adolescent men and women about these gendered significations.

A fundamental claim underpinning the notion of the gendered space is that situations of change need to be elaborated *and* brought about by the interested parties themselves, if transformations are to stand a stronger chance of being locally acceptable and of having a sustainable impact on the social fabric of the community (Freire 1972, 1976, 1997). The gendered space, as a conceptual tool, is based on the assumption that the generation of a sphere that hosts a change-enabling environment can help the community to facilitate open communication, promote social action, and enact sensitive transformations.

The notion of gendered space attempts to capture two key issues that are fundamental in the process of generating sustainable community transformation. First, the gendered space emerges from within the resources available in the community. It is, from its inception, a fully local sphere embedded in local practices. The community at large operates as a permanent partner in interaction with the gendered space. Every step accomplished within the gendered space is subjected to validation by the community. In short, the gendered space is rooted in the community itself, constantly and unavoidably relating to it. Second, the gendered space is always inhabited by local members. Born and bred locally, the gendered space is also locally owned. It provides a forum for expression, interaction and exchange where emotional, as much as cognitive, considerations affect and effect social action. Social action in turn becomes the very achievement of the gendered space, the point of contact that links the agents of gendered spaces to the community, that transforms existing resources into new ones, and blends continuity and change.

As such, the gendered space can be seen in terms of two sets of relations that provide the lifeblood to its existence, and make the act of negotiation an inextricable part of its substance. On the one hand, the gendered space is moulded and shaped by its relations with the community's social agents. On the other hand, the gendered space, as an arena for interaction and experience, is enacted by relations among the participants of this space. These two sets of relations produce in the gendered space a positive pressure that invites, promotes and induces innovation and creativity. A pressure that elicits the community's identity, as much as it facilitates the unfolding of individual agency. It is a pressure which provides the catalyst for change.

However, the gendered space, as a conceptual tool, needs to be understood both in relation to the actual promotion of sexual health, and within a framework of practical implementation. These two issues will be addressed in the next sections. First, we will show how the notion of gendered space can shed light on adolescent sexual health promotion. Next, we will illustrate how we implemented the notion of gendered spaces by setting up 'adolescent networks', loose organisational arrangements that bring together young women and men to realise social activities in the community.

Gendered spaces as arenas for sexual health promotion

Past attempts in sexual health promotion have tended to focus on the 'content' of personal decisions regarding sexual behaviour: how our reproductive system works, what biological risks are involved, what contraceptive methods are available and where to find them, etc. Little has been said, and even less has been done, to address the fact that, more than individual calculations about biology, risks and related technologies, decisions regarding sexual health are inherently and fundamentally shared decisions. Indeed, it is crucial that sexual health promotion take this basal *intersubjective* aspect of sexuality into account and act to facilitate the sharing of the decision-making process (Habermas 1987). This necessarily involves considerably more than providing information for the egocentric calculations of isolated individuals striving for self-efficacy. Shared decisions require, by definition, that interactions be characterised by an awareness and consideration of others' subjectivity.

Incorporating these crucial issues into adolescent sexual health promotion requires that the social context of the decision-making process and the shared nature of decisions be fully acknowledged by promotion initiatives. More importantly, however, it requires that these be openly *elaborated and exercised* by the adolescents themselves. It requires that careful effort be dedicated to the generation of possibilities for *open* discussion that is not bound by conflicting institutional constraints, as is the case in many school- or hospital-based projects (UNFPA 1997). Above all, it requires that a bold stress be put on the *processes* of elaboration and exercise, by subjects, of their own understandings and actions; rather than on decontextualised outcomes, emptied of meaningful subjective experience (Barnes *et al.* 1997, 1999).

In this context, the gendered space has been devised as a lacuna for reform – for negotiation and re-creation. It aims to establish a community-based arena for the facilitation of shared decisions, and it achieves this via the intersubjective quality of the relationships it foments.

Intersubjectivity has been given a central place in the gendered space as a means of calling attention to the power relations that are enacted in every social, and sexual, exchange (Foucault 1981, 1987). This refers not only to instances where the existence of social hierarchies leads to abuses of power and impositions of will (e.g. harassment, violence, rape, etc.), but also to the ceaseless possibility for dialogue and negotiation. As such, the gendered space is one where this possibility for interchange, where the potential for fruitful communication, is exploited to a maximum, so that interaction is characterised by subject/subject relations, in favour of subject/object regimes. In subject/subject relationships the scope of the decision process is broadened from self-centred interests to mediated considerations that privilege negotiation, dialogue and solidarity. In turn, such interactions demand that the focus of attention shift from the adult's version of propriety, to the adolescents', privileging their creativity and ownership in the inevitable, daily reconstruction of their life-world (Habermas 1987).

Indeed, this reconstruction of the life-world is paramount in the nourishment of a gendered space, where the apparently natural character of internalised patterns is challenged and 'historised', and identities are re-created (Attride-Stirling 1998). However, the community, the immediate society, remains the anchor for this process of challenge and re-creation, and while the founding principles of the culture will be questioned and reassessed, this will always take place within the culture's own discourses, contradictions and parameters. As such, the gendered space remains embedded in the culture, a part of its community and a catalyst for changes that are locally desired. Local sensitivity and acceptability are, indeed, crucial qualities of the gendered space, and it is precisely this that is its most distinctive strength: the precariousness of its boundaries. It sits inside the culture and instigates challenge and debate from within the community's parameters. It creates an internal reformation, while reinforcing the community's resilience.

Health, as a resource for living (WHO 1981, 1982, 1986, 1993, Bankowsky *et al.* 1997) is central in this process; and sexual health, in particular, is the focus of attention. By creating a gendered space within the community the potential for internal reform is activated through the facilitation of shared decisions. The young women and men of the community create a forum for debate, interact with social agents, engage in the exchange of resources and promote, quite fortuitously, relations that are intersubjective; relations where there is dialogue and negotiation; relations where decisions are shared. The subject/subject quality of the interactions they foment thus comes to replace the more oppressive and repressive aspect of the available discourses on sex. In this way sexual health ceases to be exclusively about reproduction and biology, and becomes a social, subjective and shared experience, where desires and objectives are mutually respected.

The SaRA initiative

SaRA, Salud Reproductiva para Adolescentes (Reproductive Health for Adolescents), is a community-based initiative aiming to promote sexual health among adolescents. It is a multi-disciplinary, action-research project taking place in Peru, developed and run jointly by the Social Psychology Department of the London School of Economics, and Peruvian NGOs and Higher Education Institutions.[2]

SaRA is managed by an international team of practitioners and researchers. The local implementation of the project is carried out largely by a group of Peruvian doctors, psychologists, obstetricians and nurses, while a London-based group of social scientists contributes mainly to the research aspects of the initiative. The project is being implemented in thirteen communities located in highly deprived rural and urban-marginal areas in the Coastal, Andean and Jungle regions of Peru.[3] SaRA operates at a grass-roots level explicitly anchored on existing community networks. Community networks are understood in the project as basic systems for securing and distributing resources among community members (Humphreys 1997, Guzmán and Pinzás 1995). Accordingly, and following WHO's 'Health for All' guidelines (WHO 1981, 1982, 1986, 1993), in SaRA health in general and sexual health in partic-

ular are understood precisely as resources for living. By working
with relevant social actors and social networks in the community,
SaRA seeks to effect positive changes in the exchange and distribution of resources, mainly adolescent sexual health, in a fashion that
is locally acceptable. The issue of local acceptability, central to
SaRA, constitutes a fundamental aspect of any initiative on health,
and yet it has been under-considered by practitioners and the literature alike.[4]

Within each of these thirteen communities SaRA has set up
networks of adolescents who have been organised with the facilitation of Co-ordinators belonging to the SaRA team. Each
adolescent network is made up of a core group of approximately
twenty-five to fifty-five boys and girls, and a periphery of additional
adolescents who partake of the initiative in a less regular way. The
balance between boys and girls is roughly even among the networks,
with a slightly higher participation of women. Participants range
between ten and nineteen years of age.

The Co-ordinators are always 'persona grata' in the community;
they necessarily belong to the society within which they are
working, have experience working with adolescents and are well
respected by the community's members and young people. In this
way, the adolescent networks (or adolescent clubs, as they are infor-
mally called) emerge from their inception as embedded in the
community and take a stance as important social agents, working
alongside other community networks. However, the role of the
Co-ordinator is one of facilitator, not of sponsor or protector.

As part of the project, the adolescent networks participate
in a series of social activities designed to nurture the network
and embed it within its community by seeking collaboration and
exchange with other social agents. In short, SaRA's social activities
constitute the prime vehicle for the generation of gendered spaces
within the adolescent networks. These activities are broadly grouped
under informal, information and economic domains. However,
these three categories have only an analytic character; in practice
they blend into each other when social activities take place.

Briefly, informal activities pertain largely to recreational ventures
enacted with the direct aim of simply having a good time. These
range from social gatherings to football games and more; and while
they are encouraged by the SaRA team, they are not subsidised by
the project. Informal activities play a crucial role in the generation
of the gendered space, in particular during the early days of the

adolescent networks. In getting together to have a good time, adolescents come to know one another, overcome fears, share ideas and, above all, they accomplish important steps in building and nurturing threads of group solidarity.

The information activities encompass all types of endeavours in which the adolescents gather to receive, produce or deliver information, mainly on issues of sexual health. The character and content of such ventures is decided by the adolescents themselves, who are supported by the Co-ordinator in obtaining assistance and collaboration from locally available resources (e.g. health professionals) in the organisation of workshops, talks, visits, etc. The broad scope and loose structure of the information activities allow for the implementation of a wide variety of projects. While the vast majority of the activities are carried out by groups of boys and girls together, some events are organised by and for more specific groups; for example, boys or girls, older adolescents or younger ones.

Last, the economic activities encompass ventures enacted by the adolescent networks with the aim of becoming self-sustainable. One of the principal goals of SaRA is to create adolescent networks that can function independently once the project has finished. To this end, the networks carry out economic activities (e.g. food stalls in the local markets, sporting events, etc.) as a means of gaining financial independence. They are aided in this task by the Co-ordinator and a Sustainable Activities Fund made available by SaRA to proposals which make sound economic sense, and promote adolescent and community participation.

Given this account of the rudimentary structure and functioning of SaRA, we show below how gendered spaces are generated and maintained within these adolescent networks or clubs. For this purpose, actual experiences taking place in the adolescent networks will be presented and interpreted, indicating how the notion of the gendered space unfolds in practice.

Gendered spaces in practice: the SaRA experience

The interface between theory and practice always highlights gaps as well as accomplishments. As mentioned earlier, SaRA is in its second year of implementation, and key issues have come to light in terms of the workings of the adolescent networks and the emergence of gendered spaces within them.

First, the initial steps towards the creation of gendered spaces were achieved by establishing adolescent networks in the communities. Public calls informing about the new networks were made jointly by the SaRA team and key community social actors. These calls were tailored to the specific local needs, and included activities such as direct talks with adolescents in schools, fliers in local shops, local radio announcements, and door-to-door techniques. The adolescent networks were set up in open encounters taking place in highly visible places, e.g. the community's main square. During these events every potentially interested party (e.g. the adolescents, their families, local leaders, etc.) was informed about the new initiative and, more importantly, was encouraged to contribute views and opinions. These procedures generated active community participation, providing the emerging adolescent networks with essential local validation, thus constituting the first steps towards the generation of gendered spaces.

Each network was assigned a Co-ordinator. In the initial stages of network creation they provided essential guidance and encouragement, particularly in delineating the parameters and objectives of SaRA. However, an effort was made at every turn to bring across an atmosphere of collaboration *with* the young people, as opposed to working *for* them or simply *giving* them things. As the networks matured, Co-ordinators became prime adult referents for them: sources of inspiration and support as much as active agents, who also engaged in processes of debate, negotiation and consensus.

This ongoing process of negotiation, at times creative, at times controversial, generated in turn other more reflexive processes. First, these extended into the network, promoting internal debate and discussion, which enhanced the possibility for the adolescents to appropriate the network. That is, active debate and negotiation contributed to the emergence of gendered spaces from within the adolescent networks. Second, these processes also extended outside the adolescent network, providing Co-ordinators with a key role in the interlocking of network and community, while at the same time preventing Co-ordinators from becoming gatekeepers.

An important consequence of these processes has been the differentiation of the adolescent networks from traditional social arenas such as the church, the school, the social club, etc. – places which are distinctly adult-owned, even if adolescents participate in them. SaRA's emphasis has been on full adolescent agency at every level, from the content and substance to the architecture and mechanisms of the networks. In the adolescent networks as gendered spaces all dynamics are fully steered by the adolescents; decisions are enacted, goals are set and actions pursued, all based on a debate conducted by the young people themselves. Indeed, many sexual health promotion programmes have been criticised for carrying an explicitly adultist agenda (Milburn 1996). In SaRA's adolescent networks, however, the agenda is freed from direct adult intervention, so that, although the young people's world necessitates interaction with adults, their activities are not limited to or by adults' prescriptions. However, adolescent networks as gendered spaces do not function as isolated arenas, but are firmly rooted in the life of their communities.

Interaction, discussion and debate emerge in the wide range of social activities (informal, information and economic) which the networks carry out in their community. Communication and social action are treated as indivisible from each other: in performing social activities in the communities, adolescents express themselves, re-creating local values and norms. It is in these very instances of open expression that the reflexive opportunity for change lies. Some examples may shed light on the actual working in practice of the adolescent networks as gendered spaces.

Example 1 – As part of the information activities, all the networks were encouraged to produce a drama about sexuality. In these exercises, the act of coming up with a story, writing a script and acting it out, presented a poignant opportunity for the adolescents to select and research a topic for a drama (e.g. teenage pregnancy), discuss possible outcomes (e.g. abortion, marriage, stigmatisation), and negotiate together on the desired moral of their story (e.g. don't have sex, don't have abortions, have sex responsibly, etc.). By working together on an activity that was as educational as it was entertaining, the networks' young men and women found themselves in an atmosphere of exchange, debate and negotiation of meanings; they found themselves in a gendered space.

'Sexuality dramas' were produced by the adolescents in video format, making use of multi-media technologies provided by SaRA. These videos were presented to the other networks in workshops. Each presentation was followed by lively and at times heated debate, in which the manifold significations of sexuality were thoroughly scrutinised by the adolescents. Thorny topics, e.g. violence (sexual, domestic, urban, etc.) and homosexuality, came to the fore in these debates. The exploration of the topics and their cultural, ethical and practical significations were vividly explored and articulated in these discussions. The gendered spaces ambition showed promising signs of potentiality.

Example 2 – As part of the economic activities, SaRA's Sustainable Activities Fund financed a project for the creation of a vegetable garden and a 'compost field' by an adolescent network from a rural village in the Central Jungle area. The network, with the support of the Co-ordinator, gained access to a piece of land next to (and owned by) the local Health Centre. In addition, by liasing with local NGOs working in the field of rural development, the network secured technical support and training for the adolescents. At the time of writing this paper, the first lots of compost were being sold by the network to local coffee growers.

This case illustrates, for example, the local root of the kind of decisions taken by the adolescents (e.g. 'let's make money by working the land'). It shows, above all, the working in practice of a gendered space: adolescents decide on what to do; they negotiate and secure the resources needed for the fulfilment of the social activity, from those that are locally available; and they carry out the agreed plans. The example also gives an indication of the simultaneous proximity and remoteness of sexual health promotion, as it is treated in SaRA. At first sight, the promotion of sexual health does not appear to be about getting together to plough the soil, or does it?

An inherently social understanding of sexual health, anchored in collective practices rather than in individual rationality, performed within socio-economic boundaries rather than in a natural vacuum, and invested with gender and history rather than sex and biology, calls attention to the multitude of voices, which lie at the heart of the everyday experience of the adolescents. As such, we consider SaRA economic activities as privileged instances for the appropriation by the adolescent of the possibilities for shaping their environment, rather than as disconnected ventures, foreign to sexual health promotion.

Example 3 – The adolescent networks as gendered spaces have also helped the boys and girls to overcome barriers of access to available health promotion resources. Some information about sexual health is locally available in nearly all of the communities in which SaRA is operating (through hospitals, health centres, etc.), but the problem is getting young people to actually go to these sources and access available services and products. By working as a collective and being in constant dialogue with other community agents, the adolescent networks have organised visits to health centres, talks with health professionals, workshops, and other activities – they have acted as gendered spaces. As a local nurse expressed, after participating in one information activity workshop with an adolescent network in the Central Andes, 'a positive aspect is certainly constituted by adolescent participation, but more important is the opportunity created for the adolescents to communicate with each other, to analyse by themselves their own problems and to look for alternatives, which will enable them to gain awareness regarding their role in society'.

Information activities, as enacted by the adolescent networks, have contributed to the improvement of the productivity of the health care infrastructure by increasing the actual use of the existing products and services; and by working as preventive measures and thus diminishing the need for medical intervention. Furthermore, these activities have also elicited awareness among the health professionals themselves by having contact with and access to interested, enthusiastic and proactive young people. In this way the impact of adolescent networks as gendered spaces has extended beyond the participating adolescents, reaching the health professionals contacted, the families of the young people, their peers, etc.

In proceeding in this manner, what we aim to emphasise is the positive aspects of available practices and discourses. Rather than telling the young people what to do or what to think (e.g. sex is bad or abortion is okay), we are creating *with* them an environment where options and alternatives can be considered in the context of their own life-worlds. Thus gendered spaces continue to regenerate and reproduce themselves in the niches of relationships between the network and health professionals, between the adolescents and their families, between the young people and their peers, thereby strengthening the community in general.

During the second year of SaRA, the project is exploiting further the emerging autonomy and established creativity of the gendered spaces in the adolescent networks. One goal is to enable some of the adolescents to become health promoters, for example, by getting the networks involved in the task of creating sexual health promotion materials (e.g. leaflets, posters, etc.). This is paramount in the internalisation by the young people of their position as social agents, and it is achievable by getting them to identify the gaps in the available services (e.g. information campaigns aimed at urban, white, middle-class people), and having them design and implement means of addressing some of these gaps (e.g. producing material that reflects the class and ethnicity of the local population). Above all, we want the gaps to be identified by the young men and women themselves, and for them to decide on ways of addressing these issues, and design ways of tackling these problems. It is in this way that we talk about exploiting the creative pressure inherent in the gendered spaces: by conceiving and making them spaces for questioning, for challenge, for dialogue, sharing and negotiation – and, above all, spaces for change. As attested by a young woman, speaking on behalf of her peers at a workshop, 'we're extremely pleased and proud to be part of SaRA; we have learned a great deal about our Peruvian communities, about our sexuality, about ourselves and, most importantly, about each other'.

Recreating and researching: the uses of multi-media technologies

In this effort to address adolescent sexual health from a novel perspective, we developed the idea of the gendered space as a medium for sexual health promotion based on participation, dialogue and negotiation, where solidarity and mutual respect characterise social interactions and facilitate shared decision processes. Accordingly, we incorporated multi-media technologies into the project with the expectation that these would both help us to capture and explore the processes at work in the unfolding of the project, and to exploit and assist SaRA's aims.

Multi-media tools play a role at every stage of the project. The adolescents, provided with paper and pencil, tape recorders and photo and video cameras, generate textual and audio-visual accounts on the life and activities of their networks. In this section we will focus on the manifold uses of multi-media in SaRA.

Multi-media technologies have three interrelated roles in SaRA. First, they are central in SaRA's research strategy, as the sensitivity afforded by these tools contributes greatly to our endeavour to understand social processes. The research we are presently conducting with the use of these technologies focuses on two specific objectives: first, to assess the emergence and workings of

the gendered space; and, second, to explore adolescents' constructions of their life-world in general, and sexual health in particular.
These aims are also being investigated with other methods, e.g.
interviews, focus groups and observation.

Second, multi-media technologies have an important role in the
emergence and maintenance of the adolescent networks as gendered
spaces, a phenomenon that is being both exploited and investigated.
In particular, these tools exert an influence in the generation of the
gendered space; the use of textual and audio-visual materials clearly
has an impact on adolescents' constructions of themselves and their
communities; and the communication and sharing of experiences
between adolescents from distant communities is definitely facilitated by these tools. We are exploring how, why and to what extent
these processes occur.

Lastly, multi-media tools play a significant role in the generation
of sexual health promotion information. Adolescent authorship in
the generation of ideas and the production and presentation of
textual and audio-visual materials, becomes a powerful mechanism
enabling adolescents to have direct involvement in the field of
sexual health promotion. This opportunity arising from the creative
use of multi-media technologies is again a resource that is both
capitalised and explored in SaRA.

These interwoven uses of multi-media, as outlined above, pose
challenges that we cannot expect to exhaust within the limits of
SaRA, and much less within the tight boundaries of this chapter.
However, the unifying thread that we wish to emphasise here is the
centrality given to adolescents' accounts, adolescents' vision and
adolescents' voice; in short, to adolescents' agency. The gendered
space provides a sphere for the exercise of agency and multi-media
tools provide an eloquent language for its articulation.

The decision to make use of multi-media technologies was based
on clear theoretical considerations. Indeed, it is precisely because we
privilege *adolescents'* elaborations and interpretations of the world
that we have made use of multi-media technologies, and the most
crucial point to be made is that *they* have the largest stake in the
production of knowledge. Multi-media tools have proved superb in
eliciting and appreciating adolescents' own sense making. Indeed,
our starting point was a conceptualisation of sexual health promotion based on facilitating negotiation processes and shared
decisions. Multi-media technologies have provided the adolescents
with a powerful language for reflection and expression, and us with

a fertile methodology for understanding and exploring the key processes at stake. But how, and to what extent, did multi-media tools play a role in practice?

Multi-media has been woven into the fabric of SaRA's implementation. All the networks have been given access to video cameras, photo cameras, tape recorders and paper and pencil. Some of the networks' members have received basic training in the use of this equipment; and they, in turn, train other adolescents in the group. Adolescents participating in the networks are thus encouraged to generate, in multi-media format, accounts of their informal, information and economic activities (e.g. a football match, a visit to a health centre or a Salsa party fundraiser). These locally generated and locally owned textual and audio-visual accounts provide a powerful source for the understanding and exploration of the unfolding of social processes and the utilisation of community resources in practice. Indeed, adolescents' social activities are SaRA's *raison d'être*; and adolescents' accounts, its best possible testimony. The following example illustrates the uses of multi-media in the field.

As mentioned in the previous section (example 1), all SaRA adolescent networks were encouraged to produce a drama about sexuality in video format. The vast majority of the networks took up this proposal as an important challenge. Lively debates took place in making decisions about what story to tell, where to film it, who would act in it, what moral it should have, etc. The adolescents were also encouraged to document the gatherings in which the drama was being realised. For this purpose they filmed themselves discussing and planning, preparing and rehearsing, indoors and outdoors, trying on outfits, etc. 'Sexuality dramas' were then presented by the authors at SaRA workshops, and each presentation was followed by a question time (which was also documented in multi-media).

The 'sexuality dramas', their realisation, presentation and discussion, provided both the research team and the adolescents with highly valuable material. Researchers collected several video-dramas together with audio-visual and textual documentation on the production of the films, as well as on their presentation and discussion. This material contains invaluable information about the working of the networks, their relationship with the communities and, above all, about the adolescents who inhabit the gendered spaces. The dramas themselves provide the researchers with first-hand access to adolescent constructions of social relationships and, more importantly, access to the way in which these constructions unfold in the community. The full stories (dramas plus the production, presentation and discussion material) provide the research team with information about the networks' activities, and about the community and its resources. They allow us to look into the adolescents' life-world and explore their meaning systems and the emergence and working of their gendered space.

The realisation of the dramas proved to be a fun, though challenging test for the gendered spaces, and an extraordinary catalyst in the motivation of social activities. The combination of multi-media tools with drama opened up a sensitive opportunity for the adolescents to articulate pressing issues related to sexuality. They found a powerful language of expression in textual and audio-visual stories. More importantly, the stories were then turned back onto the adolescents, aiding reflection, and re-shaping and moulding their understanding of themselves. As such, multi-media tools have contributed to SaRA's goal of generating gendered spaces, while helping the adolescents to improve their communicative skills and competence. Moreover, presenting and discussing the dramas opened up a fertile space for the sharing of experiences between adolescent from different, and often isolated, communities. Above all, however, they provided a space for reflection.

Finally, some closing remarks on the uses of multi-media technologies. The tools were brought into the project with the aim of benefiting the adolescents as much as the SaRA team. Indeed, they have proved to be a fun way of instigating and articulating adolescent participation. Multi-media tools have also helped us in our research endeavour, as they have proved to be permeable to the manifold interconnections of complex processes at stake in SaRA. At present we are developing plans to exploit the richness of this textual and audio-visual information further. In particular, we are aiming to produce adolescent sexual health promotion information that can reach a wide audience through CD-ROMs, the Internet, television, etc. The road to fulfilling this ambitious goal is not without obstacles and challenges. Nevertheless, multi-media technologies have shown promising signs of potentiality; and above all, they have proved to be an inspiring source of motivation.

Conclusion

The notion of the gendered space, as put into practice in SaRA, is a project in progress, and only preliminary observations can be provided at present. However, these indicate that there is clear promise in the work being carried out and, most importantly, that the issue of adolescent sexual health promotion is being tackled in a novel and fruitful way.

Our prerogatives in SaRA have been, first, to emphasise the cultural sensitivity of the approach by rooting all the work in community networks; second, to overcome the problem of the adultist agendas that pervade initiatives targeting adolescents, by creating arenas for adolescent ownership of a gendered space; and, third, to bring to the forefront of the agenda the concerns of the adolescents themselves, by giving them the motivation and the tools to tell us their perspective. A cursory glance at the difficulties that arise from the lack of consideration of adolescents' points of view proves that there is simply little understanding and information available on the way in which adolescents construct sexuality, and how best to work with and exploit their willingness to explore these issues. As a sad consequence, adolescents are all too often neglected by policy-makers and project developers and, when there is the intention of considering and involving them, there is very little knowledge as to what to do.

We have proposed the notion of the gendered space as a sphere to be appropriated by the adolescents; an arena that enables and promotes discussion, dialogue and negotiation both among themselves, and within their communities. The SaRA adolescent networks that succeeded in creating gendered spaces, showed clear signs of collective agency, organising and carrying out a wide range of social activities. Moreover, it is already clear that the stories in multi-media format have actively involved the adolescents in promoting sexual health. In addition, they have proved powerful tools for understanding adolescent concerns and for gathering information about adolescents' perspectives.

These early positive signs of the functioning of the gendered spaces in the field have come hand in hand with an array of difficulties. SaRA's zealous concern with adolescent agency and community acceptability pose challenging questions: How is the relationship between the community and the 'outside team' built? Who sets the agenda? How are project's turns and exceptions handled? Does anyone know best? What constitutes adequate evaluation criteria? These are among the many issues that impact directly on SaRA and reach deeply into the heart of both theory and practice. The world of the adolescent is an adult design, and 'developing' countries' interventions are 'developed' countries' designs. SaRA faces the challenges raised by these problematic realities in its endeavour to contribute to the promotion of adolescent sexual health – yet another area mined with controversy. The project has put into practice the notion of gendered spaces, retreating its agenda to the implementation of substantive procedures that promote adolescent participation and community solidarity. As such, in its short history SaRA has managed to build local pockets of transformation which, although venturous in progress, already show promising signs.

The future of SaRA is promising in terms of both implementation and research. The emerging autonomy and creativity of the adolescent networks give every indication that these are, in fact, spaces for interaction, exchange and solidarity. Indeed, the emerging gendered spaces are already proving a challenge to traditional approaches to sexual health promotion with young people. As the networks mature and settle into their communities' daily existence, their relationship with the project team and other community networks should evolve, metamorphosing more and more into a relationship of co-operation and exchange. Thus, the adolescents should cease to be constructed as 'the Other', and their sexuality will cease to be conceived as a force to be controlled and suppressed by us.

Acknowledgements

This project is funded by the Department for International Development of the United Kingdom (Innovation Fund Grant AG1035, Project SaRA – Salud Reproductiva para Adolescentes/ Reproductive Health for Adolescents). However, the Department for International Development can accept no responsibility for any information provided or views expressed.

Notes

1   There are many examples of this: see for instance OMS (1989, 1993) or Maddaleno *et al.* (1995); see CEDER (1992), Sobrevilla and Cáceres (1993), Gonzales (1994), La Rosa (1995), MINSA (1996) or Salazar Cóndor *et al.* (1996) for particular references to Peruvian adolescents;

see Milburn (1996) for a critical review of initiatives which fail to consider adolescents' perspective. For a theoretical conceptualisation of the problem of excluding the voice of the affected parties, see Freire (1972, 1997); and for enlightening examples of this issue, see Habermas (1994, 1996).

2   SaRA is part of the 'Children by Choice, not Chance' initiative launched in 1991 by the UK's Overseas Development Administration (ODA) (in May 1997 the ODA disappeared; in its place, the Department for International Development (DFID) was created). The initiative focused on 'enabling millions of people to have children *by choice, not chance* and to benefit from better health' (ODA 1995: 2). As part of the implementation strategy of the 'Children by Choice' initiative, the ODA set up the Seedcorn Fund (now Innovation Fund), for funding innovative interventions in reproductive health; it identified 'adolescents' as a priority group. The UK/Peruvian team that developed SaRA took up the focus on choice and agency as promoted by ODA, and devised a community-based intervention programme grounded on adolescent choice (the emphasis being on the ODA's notion of choice, to a greater extent than on the ODA's notion of *adolescent*, which is a highly problematic concept in a context like the Peruvian communities where SaRA operates). Moreover, the Seedcorn Logical Framework set ample scope for determining the categories against which to assess project successes. This enabled the SaRA team to fully incorporate the Peruvian adolescents into every stage of the development of the project and to operate within a wider conceptualisation of sexual health promotion. The result was a project in which both adults and adolescents participate and decide on the course of the intervention.

3   The thirteen communities are distributed as follows: six in the Department of Ayacucho, in the Southern Andes; four in the Department of Junín, in the Centre of Peru; one in the Department of Ica, in the Coastal Region; and one in the Province of Callao, in the Coastal Region. The Ayacucho communities are the rural villages of Cangallo, Muruncancha and Coracora, and the urban-marginal communities of Carmen Alto, Vista Alegre and Artesanos (all three located in the fringes of the city of Huamanga). The Junín communities are the rural Andean villages of Chupaca and Paccha, the rural Jungle village of San Martín de Pangoa, and the urban-marginal community of La Victoria (on the outskirts of the city of Huancayo). Ica's community is the rural village of El Carmen. Last, Callao's is the urban-marginal community of Gambeta/Santa Rosa.

4   The importance of local acceptability has been an issue consistently raised by practitioners (see Freire (1972, 1976) for a comprehensive analysis of the problem; and see Pauccar Meza *et al.* (1990), Palomino (1993), and Meentzen (1993) for interesting Peruvian examples on how feminist informed approaches can tackle the pressing issue of local acceptability in practice).

References

Atkin L., Ehrenfeld N., Pick S. (1996) 'Sexualidad y fecundidad adolescente'. In: A. Langer, K. Tolbert (eds) *Mujer: Sexualidad y Salud Reproductiva en México*. Mexico: Edamex and The Population Council.

Attride-Stirling J. (1998) *'Becoming natural: an exploration of the naturalisation of marriage'*. Unpublished Ph.D. Thesis, University of London.

Bankowsky Z., Bryant J., Gallagher J. (eds) (1997) *Ethics, Equity and the Renewal of WHO's Health for All Strategy: Proceedings of the XXIXth CIOMS Conference*. Geneva: Council for International Organisations of Medical Sciences.

Barnes J., Stein A., Rosenberg W. (1997) 'Evidence-based medicine and child mental health services'. *Children and Society*. 11: 89–96.

—— (1999) 'Evidence based medicine and evaluation of mental health services: methodological issues and future directions'. *Archives of Diseases in Childhood*. 80: 280–5.

CEDER (Centro de Estudios para el Desarrollo Regional) (1992) *Educación Sexual para Adolescentes*. Arequipa: Centro de Estudios para el Desarrollo Regional.

Collier R. (1995) *Masculinity, Law and the Family*. London: Routledge.

Foucault M. (1981) *The History of Sexuality Volume 1: An Introduction*. Harmondsworth: Penguin.

—— (1987) 'The ethic of care for the self as a practice of freedom'. In: J. Bernauer, D. Rasmussen (eds) *The Final Foucault*. Cambridge, MA: MIT Press.

Freire P. (1972) *Pedagogy of the Oppressed*. London: Sheed and Ward.

—— (1976) *Education, the Practice of Freedom*. London: Writers and Readers Publishing Cooperative.

—— (1997) 'A response'. In: P. Freire, W. Fraser, D. Macedo, T. McKinnon, T. Stokes (eds) *Mentoring the Mentor: a Critical Dialogue with Paulo Freire*. New York: Peter Lang.

Gonzales G. (ed.) (1994) *La Adolescencia en el Perú*. Lima: Universidad Peruana Cayetano Heredia.

Griffin C. (1993) *Representations of Youth: The Study of Youth and Adolescence in Britain and America*. Cambridge: Polity.

Guzmán V., Pinzás A. (1995) *Biografías Compartidas: Redes Sociales en Lima*. Lima: Flora Tristán Ediciones.

Habermas J. (1987) *The Theory of Communicative Action Volume 2: Lifeworld and System: A Critique of Functionalist Reason*. Cambridge: Polity.

—— (1994) 'What theories can accomplish – and what they can't'. In: M. Pensky (ed.) *The Past as Future*. Cambridge: Polity.

—— (1996) *Between Facts and Norms: Contributions to a Discourse Theory of Law and Democracy*. Cambridge: Polity.

Humphreys P. (1997) 'Networking for health'. In: A. Ritsotakis (ed.) *Networking for Health*. Copenhagen: World Health Organization.

La Rosa L. (1995) *La Salud Sexual de los Adolescentes y Jóvenes en el Perú*. Lima: Universidad Peruana Cayetano Heredia.

Maddaleno M., Munist M., Serrano C., Silber T., Suárez Ojeda E., Yunes J. (eds) (1995) *La Salud del Joven y del Adolescente*. Washington: Organización Panamericana de la Salud.

Meentzen A. (1993) *Entre la Experiencia y la Ciencia: la Igualdad en la Diversidad. Manual de Promotores de Proyectos con Mujeres Rurales*. Lima: Flora Tristán Ediciones.

Milburn K. (1996) *Peer Education, Young People and Sexual Health: A Critical Review*. Edinburgh: Health Education Board for Scotland.

MINSA (Ministerio de Salud del Perú) (1996) *Programa de Salud Escolar y del Adolescente*. Lima: Boletín MINSA.

ODA (Overseas Development Administration) (1995) *Children by Choice, not Chance: Meeting the Challenge*. London: ODA.

OMS (Organización Mundial de la Salud) (1989) *Higiene de la Reproducción en la Adolescencia: Estrategia de Acción*. Geneva: OMS.

—— (1993) *Capacitación para Orientar Adolescentes en Sexualidad y Salud Reproductiva: Guía para Facilitadores*. Geneva: OMS.

Palomino N. (1993) *Sexualidad y Salud: Una Metodolgía Educativa para Mujeres*. Lima: Flora Tristán Ediciones.

Pauccar Meza N., Salazar Segovia R., Prevost T., Reilly F. (1990) *Aprendiendo Juntas Defendamos Nuestra Salud: Una Investigación Participativa Sobre la Salud de las Mujeres de los Sectores Populares de Cusco*. Cusco: Centro Amauta de Estudios y Promoción de la Mujer.

Salazar Cóndor V., Chirinos Cáceres J., Reátegui Herrera L., Bardales Mendoza O., Alarista Flor M., Gallegos Gallegos D. (1996) *Caminemos Juntos hacia una Sexualdad Integral con Afectividad Autonomía y Respeto: Manual para Educadores en Sexualidad*. Lima: Universidad Peruana Cayetano Heredia.

Senderowitz J. (1995) *Adolescent Health: Reassessing the Passage to Adulthood*. Washington: The World Bank.

Sobrevilla L., Cáceres C. (eds) (1993) *Sexualidad Humana: Manual para Educadores y Profesionales en Salud*. Lima: Universidad Peruana Cayetano Heredia.

UNFPA (United Nations Population Fund) (1997) *Thematic Evaluation of Adolescent Reproductive Health Programmes*. New York: UNFPA.

WHO (World Health Organisation) (1981) *Global Strategy for Health for All by the Year 2000*. Geneva: WHO.

—— (1982) *Plan of Action for Implementing the Global Strategy for Health for All*. Geneva: WHO.

—— (1986) *Young People's Health: A Challenge for Society. Report of a WHO Study Group on Young People and 'Health for All by the Year 2000'.* Geneva: WHO.

—— (1993) *Implementation of the Global Strategy for Health for All by the Year 2000: Second Evaluation.* Geneva: WHO.

Chapter 10

A theoretically based, cross-cultural study of infant feeding in new mothers and their partners

Vivien Swanson and Kevin Power

Introduction

Breast-feeding has clear benefits for the developmental health of the infant (World Health Organization 1989, Campbell and Jones 1996) and has been associated with reduced infant mortality, reduced risk of auto-immune disease, and enhanced immunity to infection (Howie *et al.* 1990, Wang and Wu 1996). In Third World countries in particular, the length of breast-feeding can have a major impact on child morbidity and mortality (Jakobsen *et al.* 1996). There is also evidence of health benefit to the mother from breast-feeding. Breast-feeding appears to be protective against pre-menopausal epithelial ovarian cancer (Siskind *et al.* 1997). Similarly breast-feeding has been associated with reduced risk of breast cancer in pre-menopausal women, although evidence for this is somewhat equivocal (Michels *et al.* 1996, Katsouyanni *et al.* 1996, Thomas and Noonan 1993). Short-term benefits for the mother include more rapid return to normal weight, and practical issues such as cost and convenience (Lawrence 1989). However, it should be noted that some of these advantages may become less relevant as standards of living improve (Lindenberg *et al.* 1990).

Despite the stated benefits, breast-feeding rates in many countries fall short of the ideal, and the promotion of breast-feeding is currently the focus of national and international concern (World Health Organization 1989, Office for National Statistics 1997). Examination of the rates for initiation of breast-feeding in different countries, as shown in Table 10.1, suggests that a significant proportion of women do not initiate breast-feeding post-natally. Breast-feeding rates in the UK, and in Scotland in particular, are among the worst in Europe (Campbell and Jones 1996).

Table 10.1   Percentage of women breast-feeding post-natally (on leaving hospital) for selected countries

Country	Year	Percentage breast-feeding
Finland	1995	98
Sweden	1987	97
Poland	1996	87
Australia	1988	84
Italy	1994	75
Greece	1986	72
England and Wales	1997	68
Holland	1995	68
USA	1997	59
France	1995	50
Scotland	1997	55
Ireland	1997	45
Malta	1995	42

Sources include: Breastfeed Scotland 1995, Helsing 1990, Network News 1997, Savino *et al.* 1994

Having started breast-feeding, there is also evidence that many women fail to maintain 'exclusive' or 'predominant' breast-feeding long enough to confer the maximum benefits for their baby or themselves (O'Campo *et al.* 1992). There is wide variation in national breast-feeding initiation rates. This variation between countries may be explained by a range of socio-economic and cultural differences, for example in levels of economic development or 'modernity', family structure, attitudes to women and religious affiliations (Beasley 1991, Yeo *et al.* 1994, Ineichen *et al.* 1997a). Benefits and sympathetic policies towards parents, including maternity and paternity leave and maternity pay may also help to make breast-feeding a more realistic option for mothers intending to return to work. The Scandinavian countries, for example, are among the most generous in their maternity/paternity provision, and currently have the highest rates of breast-feeding initiation and maintenance, although this was not always the case. In Finland an intensive media campaign in the 1980s and 1990s facilitated change from a primarily 'bottle-feeding culture' to one where 98 per cent of new mothers currently breastfeed (Breastfeed Scotland 1995). Although in general, southern European countries have lower breast-feeding rates than those in northern Europe, rates are very variable within countries. In Greece, for example, breast-feeding rates are generally lower in urban than in rural areas (Matsaniotis *et al.* 1987, Fitanidis 1980, Fotiou *et al.* 1990). Breast-feeding rates also vary between different ethnic and cultural groupings within countries (Sweeney and Gulino 1987, System Three Scotland 1994, Visness and Kennedy 1997). A study by Ineichen *et al.* (1997a) noted that Jewish mothers in London were twice as likely to be breast-feeding at four to six weeks than women in other ethnic groups. However, in Ineichen's study as in others, problems arise in accurately comparing measurement of feeding behaviour at different points in time from birth to weaning. There may also be confusion regarding levels of exclusivity of breast-feeding, which may lead to confusion in comparing feeding rates between countries and cultures (*Network News* 1997).

Many studies have considered biological, social and psychological factors which might influence attitudes towards breast-feeding and bottle-feeding and infant feeding decisions. Individual characteristics of the mother, including demographic variables (e.g. age, income and education level), personality variables (e.g. introversion/extraversion, level of self-esteem and locus of control), psychological factors such as level of anxiety and depression, circumstances surrounding the birth, and general standard of health and well-being are all factors which may predict feeding intentions and behaviour (Wright *et al.* 1983, Fitzpatrick *et al.* 1994, Lawson and Tulloch 1995, Visness and Kennedy 1997). Similarly, social and cultural norms related to breast-feeding, including views of social referents (e.g. the woman's spouse or partner, her own mother, friends, and health professionals) and the perceived views of 'people in general' may influence a woman's feeding decision (Beeken and Waterston 1992, Howard *et al.* 1993, Giugliani *et al.* 1994, Littman *et al.* 1994, Barnett *et al.* 1995).

Much previous research into infant feeding behaviour has been largely descriptive and atheoretical, concentrating on the demographic and epidemiological correlates of infant feeding. Although this approach allows us to identify general factors associated with breast or bottle-feeding, it fails to take account of individual determinants of feeding intentions and behaviour. A useful approach to the study of why individuals carry out, or fail to carry out particular health behaviours has been adopted in psychological studies based on social cognition models of health behaviour. Such theoretically based models, including the Health Belief Model (e.g. Rosenstock *et al.* 1988), and the Theories of Reasoned Action and

Planned Behaviour (e.g. Ajzen 1991) have aimed to understand and identify factors, including attitudes, norms and control beliefs, which successfully predict both positive and negative aspects of health behaviour, and the relationship between behavioural intention and the performance of actual behaviours.

The Health Belief Model (HBM), for example, has enabled identification of individual perceived susceptibility to health problems, perceived severity of the problem, the costs and benefits of healthy behaviours and the role of 'cues to action', which may be internal or external to the individual, in initiating and maintaining such behaviours. The HBM has been widely applied to such behaviours as healthy eating, compliance with vaccination uptake and screening programmes, and risk behaviours such as smoking, alcohol and condom use. However, this model has been criticised for placing too much emphasis on the individual, neglecting the social context, and for adopting an over-rational view of the individual as an 'information processor', failing to take account of the role of feelings or emotions in health behaviour.

The Theory of Planned Behaviour (TPB) goes some way towards addressing these criticisms by assessing 'subjective norms' and evaluations of the views of significant others towards the target behaviour, setting behaviours in a social context, and taking account of 'irrational' views. The TPB also takes account of the influence of previous experience of the behaviour in question by assessing an individual's perceived behavioural control, i.e. whether they feel they 'can' perform the behaviour, and how easy or difficult this will be. This model has previously been successfully applied to a variety of health behaviours including exercise, dietary behaviour and breast self-examination, although the combined components of the model generally predict a greater proportion of variance in behavioural intention than in the performance of the behaviour itself.

Such models have added to understanding of several areas of health behaviours. Social cognition models may also be practically useful to health educators in identifying the relative importance of specific beliefs and attitudes for different groups of individuals, which can then be targeted in attempts to change such behaviours.

Despite their usefulness in explaining health behaviours, few studies have applied social cognition models to infant feeding intentions and behaviour, and those which have done so have failed to integrate wider social norms or cultural comparisons into the model

(Manstead *et al.* 1983, Sweeney and Gulino 1987, O'Campo *et al.* 1992). The current research intended to develop a comprehensive psycho-social model to predict infant feeding behaviour applicable in different cultural settings, and to indicate specific points at which intervention to change feeding intentions or behaviour might be targeted.

The present study was constructed to develop and test the usefulness of a social cognition-based theoretical approach to infant feeding behaviour to be applied in cross-cultural settings. The primary aim was to examine the relationship between feeding beliefs, normative values, perceived behavioural control, feeding intention and infant feeding behaviour in new mothers and their partners, in urban and rural hospital settings in Scotland. A secondary aim was to carry out a cross-cultural comparison of attitudes, utilising data from a small pilot sample of new mothers and their partners in Greece. Both countries have relatively low initiation rates of breast-feeding in comparison with Scandinavian countries, although available statistics suggest that Greece has slightly higher rates than Scotland overall (Matsaniotis *et al.* 1987).

Methods

A sample of 203 mothers who had given birth in the previous forty-eight hours were recruited over a three-month period in two hospitals in Scotland, one in the urbanised central belt and another in the more rural Highland Region. The women were interviewed by independent postgraduate researchers using a semi-structured questionnaire. Interviews were voluntary and confidential. All primiparous and multiparous mothers experiencing 'normal' vaginal or caesarean section delivery of babies during the three-month study period were eligible for inclusion. Following interview, mothers were given a questionnaire to be completed by their partner and returned to researchers in a pre-paid envelope. An identical procedure was followed for the pilot study in Greece. A sample of twenty-five mothers was recruited from two city hospitals in Athens, and interviewed by a postgraduate researcher within forty-eight hours of delivery. Their partners were also given a questionnaire to return by post.

The same interview procedure and questionnaires were used in both Scottish and Greek samples.

Demographic information

Age, education level (measured on a five-point scale from 'no quali-fications' to 'degree'), employment status, marital status, housing type and details of number of previous children and feeding method were ascertained for mother and partner.

Women were asked how they had intended to feed their baby before birth (breast, bottle or combined feeding), when this feeding decision had been reached, and how they were feeding their baby in hospital at present. On the basis of the latter question, they were classified as 'breast-feeding', 'combined feeding' or 'bottle-feeding' for analysis. Definitions of breast-feeding, bottle-feeding and combined feeding in the current study were based on those used in the WHO Global Data Bank on Breast-feeding, as follows:

- *Breast-feeding*: infant receives only breast milk (including ex-pressed milk).
- *Combined feeding*: infant receives breast milk and regular bottle-feeding with baby formula milk.
- *Bottle-feeding*: infant receives baby formula milk from a bottle.

Women were also asked whether they had breastfed previous children, if applicable.

Social cognition model components

Feeding beliefs

A twenty-item feeding beliefs scale was administered. The twenty items were subsequently categorised into four subscales of five items each, measuring positive and negative beliefs about breast-feeding and bottle-feeding. Each belief item was rated on a seven-point Likert scale from 1 (disagree strongly) to 7 (agree strongly). Subscale scores therefore had a minimum value of 5 and a maximum value of 35.

Twelve of these items were derived from research by Manstead *et al.* (1983), and an additional eight items were added following a review of relevant literature. These additional items included: ease of returning to work for the mother; perception of breast-feeding as 'natural' and bottle-feeding as 'not natural'; changes to mothers' breasts as a result of breast-feeding; bottlefed babies being easier to settle; bottlefed babies putting on weight more quickly; and breast-feeding being uncomfortable for the mother. A copy of the Feeding Beliefs Scale is shown in the Appendix to this chapter. Examples of categorisation of beliefs were: 'breast-feeding protects the baby against infection' (breast-feeding (BF) positive); 'breast-feeding is embarrassing for the mother' (BF negative); 'bottlefed babies put on weight quickly' (bottle-feeding (BO) positive); 'preparing feeds for bottlefed babies is inconvenient' (BO negative).

Social norms

These were measured by recording level of agreement/disagreement with statements about social referents' views regarding infant feeding, also based on Manstead *et al.*'s (1983) research. There were five statements each regarding breast-feeding and bottle-feeding, for example, 'my midwife(s) think I ... ' varying only in the named social referent. As in Manstead *et al.*'s paper, referents were the baby's father, own mother, closest female friend, and midwives. However for the present study, normative agreement with people at greater social distance, i.e. 'people in general' was also measured. This item was worded 'people in general think that women ... '. The seven-point Likert response scale had end points labelled 'definitely should not breastfeed/bottlefeed' (1), and 'definitely should breastfeed/bottlefeed '(7).

Evaluations

The importance of each referent's views was also evaluated. An example was: 'people in general's views on feeding babies are ... '. This seven-point scale had end points labelled 'not at all important to me' (1) and 'very important to me' (7). Infant feeding beliefs scales were completed by mothers and their partners. Social normative items and evaluations were completed by mothers only.

Perceived control over infant feeding method

This was also rated, first, in respect of the decision made before birth, and second, regarding the feeding decision in hospital by two items: i.e. 'how much control do you feel you had over this decision about feeding your baby' (a) before birth and (b) in hospital. Seven point Likert scales, with end points representing 'complete control' (1) and 'no control' (7), were utilised.

Breast-feeding and bottle-feeding mothers in the Scottish sample, and breast-feeding and combined feeding mothers in the Greek sample were compared in terms of their responses to the above items using chi square analysis for categorical data and t-tests for continuous data. A hierarchical regression analysis was used to determine which of the components of the Theory of Planned Behaviour social cognition model were most useful in predicting breast-feeding in hospital for the Scottish sample.

Results

A total of 203 mothers and 99 partners completed questionnaires in the Scottish study. The response rate for partners (based on the number of mothers currently living with partners) was 53 per cent. A total of 25 mothers were included in the Greek study, and 12 partners responded (partners' response rate 52 per cent). It is acknowledged that the numbers in the Greek study were relatively small, and conclusions based on comparisons of this sample with the larger Scottish sample should be treated with caution.

Demographic comparisons

Statistical comparisons revealed few significant differences between mothers from hospitals in Central and Highland Regions in Scotland in terms of demographic characteristics, feeding beliefs or norms, so these groups were combined for the analysis. Although mothers and partners in the Greek sample were slightly older than those in Scotland, the sample profiles were similar in terms of marital status, housing tenure and parity, as shown in Table 10.2. They were also similar in terms of mean level of education. Similar proportions of mothers were previously employed (69 per cent of Scottish sample, 60 per cent of Greek sample). Cross-cultural comparisons in terms of socio-economic group (SEG) require careful consideration, since such groupings are the product of social, political and economic factors particular to each country (Glover 1996). Unfortunately insufficient information was available to us to make accurate socio-economic comparisons for this study.

In hospital at time of interview, 122 (60 per cent) mothers in the Scottish sample were exclusively breast-feeding, seventy-six (38 per cent) were exclusively bottle-feeding and four (2 per cent) were combined feeding. Subsequent analysis was carried out for this

Table 10.2 Characteristics of mothers and their partners in the Scottish and Greek samples

	Scotland		Greece	
	Mothers (n = 203)	Partners (n = 99)	Mothers (n = 25)	Partners (n = 12)
Mean age (SD)	28.4 (5.8)	31.7 (5.4)	31.0 (5.5)	33.6 (5.3)
Married/ cohabiting	169 (83.3%)		25 (100%)	
Living with partner	187 (92%)		23 (92%)	
Own housing	115 (57%)		15 (60%)	
Other children	99 (49%)		11 (44%)	
Employed pre-birth	140 (69%)		15 (60%)	

sample comparing breastfeeders and bottlefeeders, excluding the small number of 'combined' feeders. Only one (4 per cent) of the mothers in the Greek sample was exclusively bottle-feeding in hospital, the majority (n = 13; 52 per cent) were 'combined' feeding and the remainder (n = 11; 44 per cent) exclusively breast-feeding. Exploratory analysis showed no statistically significant differences between the breastfeeders and combined feeders in the Greek sample, in terms of demographic characteristics (age, education level, etc.), mother's or partner's infant feeding beliefs or mother's subjective norms. This sample was therefore treated as one group for comparison with breast-feeding and bottle-feeding mothers in the Scottish sample.

When breastfeeders and bottlefeeders in the Scottish sample were compared in terms of the above demographic characteristics, bottle-feeders were found to be younger (mean age 26.5 years) than breastfeeders (mean age 29.7) (t = 3.9, df = 196, p<0.001), had a lower level of education (t = 6.7, df = 195, p<0.001), were less likely to be in regular employment in the year before the baby's birth (χ^2 = 5.7, df = 1, p<0.05), were of lower SEG (based on mother's employment) (t = 5.4, df = 134, p<0.01), were more likely to live in rented accommodation (χ^2 = 26.8, df = 2, p<0.001) and to be a single parent (χ^2 = 10.7, df = 2, p<0.01) than breastfeeders.

Infant feeding decision before birth

When asked about the way they had intended to feed their babies *before* birth, 130 (64 per cent) of the Scottish sample said they intended to breastfeed, seventy intended to bottlefeed and three (1.5 per cent) combine feed. A greater proportion of mothers in the Greek sample (n = 19; 79 per cent) had intended to breastfeed, none intended to bottlefeed and five (21 per cent) intended to combined feed (1 did not respond) (χ^2 = 31.8, df = 2, p<0.001). For most mothers the feeding decision was made at an early stage, seventy seven (38 per cent) of the Scottish sample made the decision pre-conception, and a further ninety-seven (49 per cent) in early pregnancy. Only twenty-two (11 per cent) made the decision in late pregnancy and six (3 per cent) after delivery. There was no significant difference between mothers breast-feeding or bottle-feeding in hospital in terms of when the feeding decision was made. In the Greek sample, most made the feeding decision at an early stage, fourteen (56 per cent) having made the decision pre-conception, although five (20 per cent) in this sample said they made the feeding decision in hospital after delivery (comparison between Scottish and Greek sample: χ^2 = 31.5, df = 3, p<0.001).

Infant feeding beliefs

The feeding beliefs of Scottish breast-feeding mothers and their partners, Scottish bottle-feeding mothers and their partners, and mothers and partners in the Greek pilot study were compared, as shown in Table 10.3.

Comparison of breastfeeders and bottlefeeders

Breast and bottlefeeders' beliefs differed significantly on three out of the four scales measuring positive and negative attitudes to breast-feeding and bottle-feeding. Mothers breast-feeding in hospital agreed more strongly with positive views about breast-feeding (t = 10.2, df = 189, p<0.001), disagreed more with positive views on bottle-feeding (t = 4.4, df = 184, p<0.001) and agreed

Table 10.3 Positive and negative breast-feeding and bottle-feeding beliefs for breast-feeding and bottle-feeding mothers and their partners in Scotland, and breast-feeding and combined-feeding mothers and their partners in Greece

	Positive breast-feeding beliefs	Negative breast-feeding beliefs	Positive bottle-feeding beliefs	Negative bottle-feeding beliefs
	mean (SD)	mean (SD)	mean (SD)	mean (SD)
Scottish breastfeeders	32.7 (2.7)	19.6 (5.8)	23.9 (4.3)	22.0 (6.9)
Scottish bottlefeeders	26.9 (5.1)	20.3 (5.8)	26.9 (4.7)	16.4 (5.3)
Scottish breastfeeders' partners	32.0 (3.0)	20.3 (5.0)	22.4 (5.0)	23.6 (6.7)
Scottish bottlefeeders' partners	25.3 (5.0)	21.9 (4.2)	25.4 (3.5)	15.0 (4.6)
Greek breastfeeders and combined feeders	32.3 (2.5)	16.3 (6.7)	25.1 (5.4)	21.0 (5.2)
Greek partners	30.5 (2.7)	18.6 (8.0)	23.9 (4.9)	24.3 (5.9)

more with negative views on bottle-feeding ($t = 5.8$, df $= 190$, $p<0.001$), than mothers who were bottle-feeding.

Comparison of feeding beliefs for mothers and their partners

Scottish breast-feeding mothers held significantly more positive beliefs about breast-feeding than their partners ($t = 2.1$, df $= 69$, $p<0.05$). However there was no significant difference between the views of breast-feeding mothers and their partners in terms of negative beliefs about breast-feeding or positive and negative bottle-feeding beliefs. Similarly Scottish bottle-feeding mothers held significantly more positive views about bottle-feeding than their partners (t = 2.2, df = 19, p<0.05). There was no significant difference between the views of bottle-feeding mothers and their partners in terms of positive and negative breast-feeding beliefs and negative bottle-feeding beliefs.

Table 10.3 also indicates that mothers and their partners in the Greek sample held views more comparable with those of the breast-feeding mothers and partners in Scotland than the bottlefeeders, although they agreed less with negative breast-feeding beliefs.[1]

Social normative beliefs

The mothers in the study indicated how far they agreed with the views of close social referents (their partner, own mother, friends), health professionals (midwives) and people at greater social distance (i.e. 'people in general') regarding breast and bottle-feeding, and also evaluated how important the views of these individuals were to them. Questions measured level of agreement/disagreement with statements such as 'my midwife thinks that I definitely should breastfeed' and evaluations of the importance of the views of each social referent. Figures 10.1a and 10.1b illustrate agreement with, and perceived importance of, the views of their partner, own mother, closest female friend, midwives, and people in general, for breast-feeding and bottle-feeding mothers in the Scottish sample, and all mothers in the Greek sample.

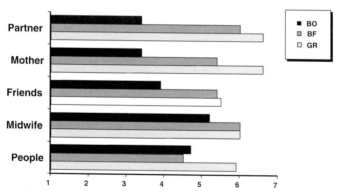

Figure 10.1a   Agreement with the breast-feeding views of partner, own mother, friends, midwives and people in general for Scottish breastfeeders, Scottish bottlefeeders, and Greek breastfeeders and combined feeders

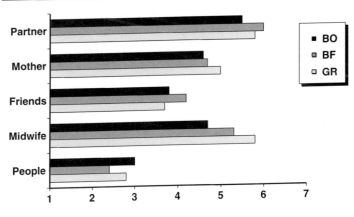

Key
BO: Scottish bottlefeeders
BF: Scottish breastfeeders
GR: Greek breastfeeders and combined feeders

Figure 10.1b   Importance of the views of partner, own mother, friends, midwives and people in general, for Scottish breastfeeders, Scottish bottlefeeders, and Greek breastfeeders and combined feeders

Agreement with social norms

For the Scottish sample, t-tests revealed that breastfeeders agreed more strongly than bottlefeeders with the views of their partner ($t = 12.9$, df = 188, $p<0.001$), own mother ($t = 8.9$, df = 188, $p<0.001$), female friends ($t = 6.6$, df = 193, $p<0.001$) and midwives ($t = 4.0$, df = 194, $p<0.001$) that they should breastfeed (an example of these questions is: 'my own mother thinks I definitely should breastfeed'). However, there was no significant difference between breast and bottlefeeders' level of agreement with the question 'people in general think women definitely should breastfeed'. Thus breastfeeders in Scotland agreed more closely with perceived social norms about breast-feeding than bottlefeeders in Scotland for their close social referents and health professionals, but not for people in general.

An identical pattern (not illustrated here) was identified for Scottish mothers in terms of agreement with social referents' views on bottle-feeding. Bottle-feeding mothers agreed more strongly than breastfeeders with their partner's views ($t = 9.8$, df = 190, $p<0.001$)

their own mother's views (t = 7.5, df = 187, p<0.001), their friends' views (t = 4.9, df = 192, p<0.001) and their midwives' views (t = 2.4, df = 194, p<0.05) that they should bottlefeed (an example of a question being 'my midwife thinks I definitely should bottlefeed'), but there was no difference between Scottish breastfeeders and bottlefeeders in terms of agreement with the normative views of people in general regarding bottle-feeding.

Breast-feeding and combined feeding mothers in Greece indicated significantly more agreement with their partner's views (t = 4.4), their own mother's views (t = 4.4) and people in general's views (t = 5.9) (all p<0.001), and with midwives' views (t = 2.8, p<0.05) about breast-feeding than bottlefeeders in Scotland, although similar comparisons with social norms of breastfeeders in Scotland for these referents were not significant. However, Greek breastfeeders and combined feeders agreed more strongly with the normative views of people in general than both breastfeeders (t = 5.8, p<0.001) and bottlefeeders in Scotland (t = 6.0, p<0.001).

Importance of the views of social referents

In terms of the relative importance of the views of other people regarding infant feeding, the views of their partners were given the highest importance rating by Scottish breastfeeders and bottlefeeders, and Greek breastfeeders and combined feeders. Figure 10.1b illustrates that, for the Scottish sample, the views of their partner (t = 2.6, df = 191, p<0.01) and their midwife (t = 2.3, df = 196, p<0.05) are significantly more important to breastfeeders than bottlefeeders. Conversely, the views of people in general are more important to bottlefeeders than to breastfeeders in this sample (t = 2.3, df = 196, p<0.05).

For breast-feeding and combined feeding mothers in the Greek sample, the infant feeding views of midwives were rated as being of equal importance to the views of their partner. Comparing the Greek and Scottish samples, the views of midwives were significantly more important for Greek mothers than for Scottish bottlefeeders (t = 5.8, p<0.001), but not Scottish breastfeeders.

Perceived behavioural control

Scottish breastfeeders (mean 1.2, SD 1.1) and bottlefeeders (mean 1.3, SD 1.2), and Greek breastfeeders and combined feeders (mean

1.4, SD 1.0) reported having a high degree of control over their feeding decision before the baby's birth, with no significant difference in amount of control between these groups. However, Scottish breastfeeders (mean 1.1, SD 0.3) reported more perceived control over their decision regarding feeding method in hospital than Scottish bottlefeeders (mean 1.3, SD 1.1) (t = 2.1, df = 195, p<0.05). (For these items, low scores represented greater perceived control.) Similarly, Greek breastfeeders reported more control over their feeding decision in hospital (mean 1.1, SD 0.3) than Greek combined feeders (mean 2.6, SD 2.1) (t = 2.2, df = 22, p<0.05), although due to the small sample size these results should be treated with caution.

Predictors of breast-feeding

Hierarchical regression analysis was carried out for the Scottish sample to determine which social cognition model components were most useful in predicting breast-feeding in hospital. Numbers in the Greek sample were too small to carry out this type of multivariate analysis. Variables were entered in blocks, first controlling for demographic differences (age, education level), second mothers' positive and negative breast and bottle-feeding beliefs, third partners' feeding beliefs, fourth social norms, and fifth perceived behavioural control and previous breast-feeding experience. Together, these variables predicted a large proportion (57 per cent) of variance in breast-feeding behaviour in hospital for the Scottish sample. Demographic variables predicted 16 per cent of variance overall, and mother's level of education was the strongest demographic predictor (beta = .24, p<0.05). Mothers' infant feeding beliefs predicted the largest amount of variance (29 per cent), and positive breast-feeding beliefs were the strongest predictor (beta = .68, p<0.001). Partners' feeding beliefs predicted a further 9 per cent of variance, with partners' positive breast-feeding beliefs being the strongest predictor (beta .30, p<0.05). Similarly the combined social norms predicted a further 9 per cent of variance, and previous breast-feeding also contributed significantly to the regression equation (beta = .20, p<0.05, 4 per cent of variance). Perceived control over the infant feeding decision did not significantly predict further variance in feeding behaviour.

Discussion

Social cognition models have been shown to be particularly useful in extending our understanding of many types of health behaviours, utilising a 'rational information processing' approach to predicting why individuals behave in certain ways (Conner and Norman 1996). By identifying particular beliefs which are important for individuals with different psycho-social characteristics, such models also have the potential to allow health professionals to specifically target interventions designed to change behaviour.

Although many studies have described characteristics of new mothers who choose to initiate breast-feeding, and some studies have previously applied components of social cognition models to infant feeding behaviour, the present study aimed to extend previous work by applying the Theory of Planned Behaviour to infant feeding behaviour. This study included the concept of perceived control over feeding behaviour, and a wider definition of social norms than has been used previously, including agreement with normative beliefs of 'people in general'. In this sense the study was perhaps unique in piloting a cross-cultural comparison of infant feeding beliefs and social norms. Health beliefs, social norms and perceived behavioural control for mothers in an urban and rural area in Scotland were compared with beliefs of Greek mothers attending two urban hospitals in Athens, Greece.

The regression analysis employed to test the Theory of Planned Behaviour suggested that mothers' positive beliefs about breast-feeding were the most important predictor of actual breast-feeding behaviour whilst still in hospital. These included beliefs that breast-feeding establishes a bond between mother and baby, that breast-feeding is natural, gives the baby the best nourishment, and protection against infection, and helps get the mother's figure back to normal. This period immediately following childbirth is very important in initiating breast-feeding behaviour. The results also emphasised that the positive breast-feeding beliefs of the woman's partner, the mother's agreement with social norms about breast and bottle-feeding, and having previously breastfed were additional significant determinants of the decision to breastfeed post-natally. Confirming findings from many other studies, this study also found that demographic factors predicted breast-feeding in hospital. Mother's level of education was the strongest demographic predictor of breast-feeding in hospital. Bottlefeeders in the Scottish sample tended to be significantly younger, have less formal education, be less likely to have been employed in the year before the birth, and to represent lower socio-economic grouping than breast-feeders. There were few significant demographic differences between mothers in Scottish urban and rural settings. Geographical location within a country may be a less important correlate of infant feeding behaviour than more specific socio-economic factors such as education level, housing tenure and occupational status.

Methodological difficulties with social cognition models are acknowledged. Such models have been criticised for neglecting key variables specific to particular health behaviours, and being static and cross-sectional rather than longitudinal and dynamic in their application (Conner and Norman 1996). There is also little evidence to date of success in actually changing beliefs, attitudes and cognitions, once they have been identified. However, social cognition models do have the advantage of providing a structured theoretical framework for research, and in this sense may be most useful if applied in conjunction with specialist knowledge of the biomedical and socio-cultural background to the health behaviour under study.

The timing of the decision to breastfeed or bottlefeed was made earlier for a larger proportion of women in this study than in other research (Fitzpatrick *et al.* 1994), with many reporting that the feeding decision was made pre-conception. Currently most knowledge-based interventions to promote breast-feeding are carried out ante-natally, during pregnancy, or following childbirth. It could be argued from these findings that school-based educational intervention, preferably before the age of sixteen, by which time attitudes towards infant feeding are likely to be formed, may be most effective in changing infant feeding behaviour, particularly since teenage mothers have been shown to be less likely to breastfeed (Ineichen *et al.* 1997b). Awareness of the benefits of breast-feeding is acknowledged as a priority for school-based dietary education in a Scottish Office report (Scottish Office Department of Health 1996). One cross-cultural study carried out in Japan and the USA found very different attitudes towards breast-feeding and its impact on family life in female high school students (Yeo *et al.* 1994). Further cross-cultural research in school-age children to determine existing levels of knowledge and specific beliefs about infant feeding related to social normative factors and the cultural context are important to ascertain the optimum age for effective intervention to improve rates of breast-feeding in the future. These questions are currently the focus of further research by the authors.

In terms of the present study, it was interesting to note that 64 per cent (130) of Scottish mothers intended before birth to breast-feed, and 60 per cent (122) of these were exclusively breast-feeding after delivery, whereas 79 per cent (nineteen) of the Greek sample intended before birth to breastfeed and only 44 per cent (eleven) of the sample were exclusively breast-feeding in hospital. Because the present study utilised a standard semi-structured interview format, we were unable to examine in depth the reasons for this gap between intentions and behaviour. A similar 'gap' is noted in many studies which aim to predict actual health behaviour from stated intentions. A different methodological approach using more qualitative open-ended questioning of responses of women whose intention to breastfeed does not match subsequent behaviour is required. One possible explanation for the discrepancy between feeding intention and behaviour in the present study is attitudes of health professionals towards breast-feeding, and the policies of the Scottish and Greek hospitals in the study regarding supplementary bottle-feeding, a factor which may be outwith the mother's own control.

Perceived behavioural control is an important component of the theory of planned behaviour which was assessed in the current study. Although perceived control was not a significant predictor of breast-feeding in the regression analysis, this may have been due to the way 'control' was assessed. 'Internal' personality factors, such as self-efficacy, self-esteem and locus of control, may influence a woman's perceived ability to initiate and continue breast-feeding as well as 'external' social, cultural, environmental or situational factors. Future studies might be improved by utilising more sophisticated measures of perceived behavioural control. It may also be more meaningful to measure control over the longer-term continuation of breast-feeding behaviour in the period following discharge from hospital, rather than control of the initiation of breast-feeding.

Breastfeeders in Scotland and Greece reported significantly more perceived control over their feeding decision in hospital than Scottish bottlefeeders and Greek combined feeders respectively. Greek mothers and Scottish breastfeeders indicated more agreement with midwives' feeding beliefs than bottlefeeders, and Greek mothers attributed more importance to midwives' views than Scottish breastfeeders and bottlefeeders. Subjective reports from the researchers who carried out the pilot study in Greece also suggest that the paediatrician generally has a more central role peri-natally in Greece than in the UK. If this role is strongly influential, Greek mothers may indeed have less control over infant feeding decisions in hospital, although individual psychological factors such as the mother's assertiveness and level of self-esteem may also be important. Several studies have also noted the importance of the role of the health professional in influencing feeding behaviour (Helsing 1990; Beeken and Waterston 1992; Howard *et al.* 1993, Barnett *et al.* 1995, Lazarro *et al.* 1995). The present study did not assess agreement with normative views of physicians as social referents. Experience with the Greek pilot study suggests that this omission should be rectified in future cross-cultural studies using this theoretical approach.

For the Scottish sample, there were clear differences between breast-feeding and bottle-feeding mothers in terms of social normative beliefs. Breast-feeding mothers agreed more strongly than bottlefeeders with the views of people close to them, their partner, mother and friends, and also with the views of midwives, about breast-feeding. They also attached more importance to the views of these individuals than did bottlefeeders. Other studies have noted that the subject's partner and their own mother generally have most influence on the feeding decision (Manstead *et al.* 1983, Sweeney and Gulino 1987, Giugliani *et al.* 1994, Ineichen *et al.* 1997b). The balance of this influence may depend on the cultural significance of the family, how 'matriarchal' the society is, and the independence of the subject from her own family. Interestingly, in the present study bottlefeeders attached more importance than breastfeeders to the views of people in general. Levels of fear of embarrassment or disapproval from others are also influenced by psychological characteristics such as extraversion, self-esteem, or assertiveness. Since breast-feeding in public or semi-public places can often attract public criticism or disapproval, this fear may be an important factor influencing bottlefeeders' decision not to breastfeed. Support from family, health professionals, or peer counsellors (Wright 1996) may be enlisted to help enhance mothers' self-confidence or self-esteem in such situations.

It is perhaps not surprising that mothers and partners hold similar views on infant feeding, although a study by Freed *et al.* (1993) reported less congruence between mothers' and partners' attitudes than the present study. In the Scottish sample, breastfeeders and their partners recorded more agreement with positive breast-feeding beliefs and negative bottle-feeding beliefs than bottlefeeders and their partners. Mothers in Greece and their partners also recorded few differences in beliefs and displayed beliefs more in common with Scottish breastfeeders than bottle feeders. Other research has noted the crucial importance of the baby's father's approval in initiating breast-feeding (Littman *et al.* 1994). The present study also had the benefit of being able to measure partners' attitudes to infant feeding directly, rather than asking for the mothers' perception of their partners' attitude which may not be an accurate reflection of his views (Freed *et al.* 1993).

It is acknowledged that this study has only made a start in identifying cross-cultural differences that predict infant feeding behaviour. The small size and geographically concentrated nature of the Greek sample of mothers and partners means that findings are not generalisable, although this exploratory study does give an indication of differences and similarities between new mothers in Scotland and Greece. A more detailed description and standardised measurement of cultural variables needs to be carried out, including examination of hospital policies and practice regarding infant feeding behaviour.

It is intended to expand the pilot study in Greece in future work, and to extend the application of the theory of planned behaviour to different cultural settings, including those with favourable and less favourable rates of breast-feeding initiation and maintenance. Following the implementation of the WHO/Unicef breast-feeding initiative, evaluation has focused on the process and policy implications of new approaches to promote breast-feeding. It is important in future to assess the impact of these changes on the individual mother, and the use of the structured social cognitive approach used in the present study provides a useful starting point for such an evaluation.

Acknowledgements

The assistance of the National School of Public Health, University of Athens with the Greek Pilot Study is gratefully acknowledged.

Note

1   Statistical analysis (t-tests) revealed significantly greater differences between the mothers in the Greek sample and Scottish bottlefeeders than between Greek mothers and Scottish breastfeeders in each case.

Appendix I   Breast and bottle-feeding beliefs

'Positive' breast-feeding beliefs[*]

- Breast-feeding protects the baby against infection
- Breast-feeding establishes a close bond between mother and baby
- Breast-feeding helps get the mother's figure back to normal
- Breast-feeding is a natural way of feeding
- Breast-feeding provides best nourishment for baby

'Negative' breast-feeding beliefs

- Breast-feeding is embarrassing for the mother
- Breast-feeding can be uncomfortable for the mother
- Breast-feeding limits the mother's social life
- Breast-feeding makes it difficult for the mother to return to work
- Breast-feeding changes the look of the mother's breasts

'Positive' bottle-feeding beliefs

- Bottle-feeding allows you to see exactly how much milk the baby has had
- Bottlefed babies are easy to settle
- Bottle-feeding makes it easier for the mother to go back to work
- Bottle-feeding makes it possible for the baby's father to be involved in feeding
- Bottlefed babies put on weight quickly

'Negative' bottle-feeding beliefs

- Bottle-feeding is not a natural way of feeding babies
- Bottle-feeding provides little protection against infection
- Bottle-feeding is a less hygienic way of feeding babies
- Bottle-feeding is an expensive method of feeding
- Preparing feeds for bottlefed babies is inconvenient

* Headings are omitted from actual questionnaire, and items presented in random order.

References

Ajzen I. (1991) 'The theory of planned behaviour'. *Organizational Behaviour and Human Decision Processes* 50: 179–211.

Barnett E., Sienkiewicz M., Roholt S. (1995) 'Beliefs about breast-feeding: a statewide survey of health professionals'. *Birth* 22: 15–20.

Beasley A. (1991) 'Breast-feeding studies: culture, biomedicine and methodology'. *Journal of Human Lactation* 7: 7–14.

Beeken S., Waterston T. (1992) 'Health service support of breast-feeding – are we practising what we preach?' *BMJ* 305: 285–7.

Breastfeed Scotland (1995) 'Student midwives study trip to Finland'. *Midwives* 108: 1,295.

Campbell H., Jones I. (1996) 'Promoting breast-feeding: a view of the current position and a proposed agenda for action in Scotland'. *Journal of Public Health Medicine* 18: 406–14.

Conner M., Norman P. (1996) *Predicting Health Behaviour*. Milton Keynes: Open University Press.

Fitanidis C. (1980) 'Incidence of breast-feeding in Nikea-Korydallos'. *Paediatriki* 43: 412–20.

Fitzpatrick C., Fitzpatrick P., Darling M. (1994) 'Factors associated with decision to breastfeed among Irish women'. *Irish Medical Journal* 87: 145–6.

Fotiou K., Tsekoura T., Savrami N. *et al.* (1990) 'Breast-feeding in Crete'. *Bulletin of the A' Paediatric Clinic, University of Athens* 37: 54–61.

Freed G., Fraley J., Schanler R. (1993) 'Accuracy of expectant mothers' predictions of fathers' attitudes towards breast-feeding'. *Journal of Family Practice* 37: 148–52.

Glover J. (1996) 'Epistemological and methodological considerations in secondary analysis'. In: L. Hantrais and S. Mangen (eds) *Cross-National Research Methods in the Social Sciences*. London: Printer.

Giugliani E., Waleska T., Vogelhut J., Witter F., Perman J. (1994). 'Effect of breast-feeding support from different sources on mothers' decisions to breastfeed'. *Journal of Human Lactation* 10: 157–61.

Helsing E. (1990) 'Supporting breast-feeding: what governments and health workers can do. European experiences'. *International Journal of Gynaecology and Obstetrics* 31 (Suppl 1): 69–76.

Howard F., Howard C., Weitzman M. (1993) 'The physician as advertiser : the unintentional discouragement of breast-feeding'. *Obstetrics and Gynaecology* 81: 1,048–51.

Howie P., Forsyth S., Ogston S., Clark A., Florey C du V. (1990) 'Protective effect of breast-feeding against infection'. *BMJ* 300: 11–16.

Ineichen B., Pierce M., Lawrenson R. (1997a) 'Jewish and Celtic attitudes to breast feeding compared'. *Midwifery* 13: 40–43.

—— (1997b) 'Teenage mothers as breastfeeders: attitudes and behaviour'. *Journal of Adolescence* 20: 505–9.

Jakobsen M.S., Sodemann M., Molbak K., Aaby P. (1996) 'Reason for termination of breastfeeding and the length of breastfeeding'. *International Journal of Epidemiology* 25(1): 115–21.

Katsouyanni K., Lipworth L., Trichopoulou A., Samoli E., Stuver S., Trichopoulos D. (1996) 'A case-control study of lactation and cancer of the breast'. *British Journal of Cancer* 73: 814–18.

Lawrence R. (1989) *Breast-feeding: A Guide for the Medical Profession*. St Lewis: Mosby.

Lawson K., Tulloch M. (1995) 'Breast-feeding duration : prenatal intentions and postnatal practices'. *Journal of Advanced Nursing* 22: 841–9.

Lazarro E., Anderson J., Auld G. (1995) 'Medical professionals' attitudes toward breast-feeding'. *Journal of Human Lactation* 11: 97–101.

Lindenberg C., Artola R., Jimenez V. (1990) 'The effect of early post-partum mother–infant contact and breast-feeding promotion on the incidence and continuation of breast-feeding'. *International Journal of Nursing Studies* 27: 179–86.

Littman H., Medendorp S., Goldfarb J. (1994) 'The decision to breastfeed. The importance of father's approval'. *Clinical Paediatrics* April: 214–18.

Manstead A., Proffitt C., Smart J. (1983) 'Predicting and understanding mothers' infant feeding intentions and behaviour: testing the theory of reasoned action'. *Journal of Personality and Social Psychology* 44: 657–71.

Michels K., Willett W., Rosner B., Manson J., Hunter D., Colditz G., Hankinson S. (1996) 'Prospective assessment of breast-feeding and breast cancer incidence among 89,887 women'. *Lancet* 347: 431–6.

Matsaniotis A., Karpathios N., Nikolaidou T., Alexaki P. (1987) 'Breast-feeding in Greece, yesterday and today'. *Bulletin of the A' Paediatric Clinic* University of Athens 34: 155–9.

Network News (1997) (Scottish Breast-feeding Network Newsletter) August.

O'Campo P., Faden R., Gielen A., Wang M. (1992) 'Prenatal factors associated with breast-feeding duration: recommendations for prenatal interventions'. *Birth* 19: 195–201.

Office for National Statistics (1997) *Breast-feeding in the United Kingdom in 1995.* London: HMSO.

Rosenstock I., Strecher V., Becker M. (1988) 'Social learning theory and the health belief model'. *Health Education Quarterly* 15: 175–83.

Savino F., Manzoni P., Tonini I., Dall'Aglio M., Tonetto P., Oggero R. (1994) 'Milk feeding of infants in the Turin district. An epidemiological survey'. *Minerva Pediatrica* 46: 261–7.

Scottish Office Department of Health (1996). *Scotland's Health, a Challenge to Us All: Eating for Health, a Diet Action Plan for Scotland.* Edinburgh: Scottish Office Department of Health.

Siskind V., Green A., Bain C., Purdie D. (1997) 'Breast-feeding, menopause and epithelial ovarian cancer'. *Epidemiology* 8: 188–91.

Sweeney M., Gulino C. (1987) 'The health belief model as an explanation for breast feeding practices in a Hispanic population'. *Advances in Nursing Science* 9: 35–50.

System Three Scotland (1994) *Breast-feeding: Report for Health Education Board for Scotland.* Edinburgh: HEBS.

Thomas D., Noonan E. (1993) 'Breast cancer and prolonged lactation. The WHO Collaborative Study of Neoplasia and Steroid Contraceptives'. *International Journal of Epidemiology* 22: 619–26.

Visness C., Kennedy K. (1997) 'Maternal employment and breast-feeding: findings from the 1988 National Maternal and Infant Health Survey'. *American Journal of Public Health* 87: 945–50.

Wang Y., Wu S. (1996) 'The effect of exclusive breast-feeding on development and incidence of infection in infants'. *Journal of Human Lactation* 12: 27–30.

World Health Organization (1989) *Protecting, Promoting and Supporting Breast-Feeding; The Special Role of Maternity Services. Joint WHO/ UNICEF statement*. Geneva: World Health Organization.

Wright J. (1996) 'Breastfeeding and deprivation: the Nottingham Peer Counselling Programme'. *MIDDIRS Midwifery Digest* 6: 212–15.

Wright H., Walker P., Webster J. (1983) 'The prediction of choice in infant feeding a study of primiparae'. *Journal of the Royal College of General Practitioners* 33: 493–7.

Yeo S., Mulholland P., Hirayama M., Breck S. (1994) 'Cultural views of breast-feeding among high-school female students in Japan and the United States : a survey'. *Journal of Human Lactation* 10: 25–30.

Chapter 11

Peer-led HIV prevention among gay men in London (the 4 gym project)

Intervention and evaluation

Jonathan Elford, Lorraine Sherr, Graham Bolding, Mark Maguire and Fraser Serle

Introduction

There is abundant evidence of continuing HIV transmission among gay men in the UK. Between 1990 and 1997, just under 1,500 new cases of HIV infection were reported each year, on average, in the UK among men who had sexual intercourse with other men. During this period, there was no evidence of a decline in the annual number of new infections reported in this group. HIV among gay men accounted for over 50 per cent of new cases reported annually in the UK throughout the 1990s – the majority in men aged twenty to thirty-nine years. Nearly three-quarters of all HIV diagnoses in gay men were reported in the south-east of England, mostly in the London area (PHLS 1998).

Risk behaviour among gay men in London

A number of studies conducted among gay men in London have reported continuing high risk sexual behaviour. Between one-third and one-half of the gay men interviewed said they had had unprotected anal intercourse in the previous six to twelve months. In the majority of cases the HIV status of the sexual partner with whom they had unprotected sex was either discordant or not known. Gay men continued to report high risk behaviour even though levels of knowledge were generally high in this group.

The Gay Men's Sexual Health Survey gathered information from 2,121 gay men (80 per cent response) using bars, clubs and GU services in London in November–December 1997. Just over 70 per cent of the men lived in inner London while the remainder lived in other parts of London and its environs. Over one-third (37 per cent) of the men reported having had unprotected anal intercourse in the previous year, the majority with a person of unknown or discordant HIV status. Overall, 19 per cent of men reported having unprotected anal intercourse with a person whose HIV status was either not known or discordant (Dodds *et al.* 1998). Findings from a survey conducted twelve months earlier among gay men in bars, clubs and GU services were similar (Nardone *et al.* 1998).

In a study conducted between September 1995 and January 1996 among people seeking an HIV test at a Same Day Testing Clinic in a London hospital (overall response 79 per cent), 285 gay men completed a questionnaire which included items on sexual risk behaviour. Of the 285 gay men surveyed, 50 per cent (143) reported unprotected anal intercourse with another man in the previous six months, the majority with a person whose HIV status was not known (Norton *et al.* 1997).

Repeated surveys were conducted among gay men resident in the UK who attended the Gay Pride festival in London in June 1993 (n = 1,620), 1994 (n = 1,753) and 1995 (n = 1,168). Over the three-year period there were no significant changes in reported sexual behaviour. In each year, approximately one-third of gay men said they had had unprotected anal intercourse with one or more partner in the previous twelve months (32.8 per cent, 31.7 per cent, 33.1 per cent for each year). Information was not available on whether the HIV status of the partner for unprotected anal intercourse was known (Hickson *et al.* 1996).

HIV prevention among gay men

The epidemiological data together with studies of sexual behaviour provide compelling evidence for the continuing transmission of HIV infection among gay men. Clearly HIV prevention remains a priority for gay men particularly in London. The challenge is to develop HIV prevention interventions that are effective. Hickson *et al.* (1996) noted that the increase in HIV prevention activities during recent years had not been matched by corresponding changes in gay men's sexual behaviour, possibly because resources had been used in a way that had had little or no impact on gay men's risk-taking.

A recent systematic review of health promotion interventions among gay men concluded that there was little well-evaluated work among this group. Of twenty-four studies which examined the impact of an intervention on attitudes, knowledge or behaviour, only five were judged to be methodologically sound (EPI Centre 1996). All five studies were carried out in North America. Criteria for soundness were that the studies included both an intervention and an equivalent control or comparison group, provided pre- and post-intervention data and reported on all relevant outcomes (Figure 11.1). The pros and cons of evaluating health promotion programmes by means of a controlled trial have been vigorously debated (Nutbeam 1998). Protagonists argue that health promotion interventions should be evaluated with the same degree of rigour as pharmaceutical drugs by means of a randomised controlled trial. Others argue that this approach restricts the evaluation to a limited range of outcome measures and ignores the processes that underline health promotion. In practice, a middle way may exist between these two extremes.

Figure 11.1   Criteria for a well-designed evaluation according to the Cochrane Collaboration (1993)

A well-designed evaluation should conform to eight method-ological principles. These are:

1   clear definition of aims
2   a description of the intervention package and design sufficiently detailed to allow replication
3   inclusion of a randomly allocated control group or a comparison group demonstrated to be equivalent to the experimental group on socio-demographic and outcome variables
4   provision of data on number of participants recruited to experimental and control groups
5   provision of pre-intervention data for experimental and control groups
6   provision of post-intervention data for experimental and control groups
7   attrition rates reported for experimental and control groups
8   findings reported for each outcome measure as described in the aims of the study

The authors of the review commented that although there had been considerable prevention work in the UK among gay men, 'much of it has been service-led and research and evaluation were at best an after-thought and at worst absent'. According to the systematic review, the use of peers and opinion leaders had been shown to be effective in the USA. The authors recommended that this approach should be further explored in well-designed evaluations in the UK.

HIV prevention using peer educators in gay bars in the USA

One of the interventions identified by the review as being both well-evaluated and effective in reducing sexual risk behaviour was by Kelly and colleagues from Wisconsin. Drawing on the diffusion of innovation model (Rogers 1983), they used peer educators to endorse HIV/AIDS risk reduction behaviour change among gay men attending bars in three small cities in Mississippi and Louisiana.

In the first study, the intervention was introduced into gay bars in one city while the other two cities served as controls (Kelly *et al.* 1991). In a second study, the intervention was introduced at intervals of three months into each of the three cities. In this way, control cities in the first phase of the study became intervention cities in the later part (Kelly *et al.* 1992). The cities were about sixty miles apart with stable, quite separate gay communities providing 'discrete, compact' environments for evaluating the intervention.

Gay men who were identified as being popular in the bars were recruited as peer educators to endorse changes in both sexual behaviour and sexual norms among other men. The peer educators were given training in how to make these endorsements and agreed to talk to a minimum of ten people about risk reduction. Surveys were conducted of men going to the gay bars in the intervention and comparison cities before the intervention, then three and six months afterwards. Information was collected on knowledge of HIV/AIDS, sexual behaviour and norms.

The proportion of men who engaged in any unprotected anal intercourse in a two-month period decreased by about one-third following the intervention. Little or no change was observed among men in the control cities over the same period of time.

Kelly *et al.* (1997) subsequently evaluated the intervention in other small towns in the USA. Peer educators were recruited and trained in gay bars in four small towns in Wisconsin, New York,

West Virginia and Washington state, while bars in four other towns in the same states (at least fifty miles away) served as controls. Questionnaires were distributed to bar patrons at baseline in all bars (intervention and control) and after twelve months. At one-year follow-up gay men in intervention towns reported a reduction in the mean frequency of unprotected anal intercourse in the previous two months – no such change was reported from the control cities.

HIV prevention using peer educators in gay bars in London

Kelly and colleagues demonstrated that peer educators can serve as agents of behaviour change in gay bars in small US cities. This may, therefore, offer a new approach to HIV prevention among gay men in the UK. Encouraging as Kelly's findings are, however, it may not be assumed that they can be directly transferred from the USA to the UK, nor from small towns to large cities such as London.

For this reason, interventions using peer educators need to be formulated and evaluated in a number of settings in the UK. If found to be effective peer-led interventions could be introduced widely by statutory and non-statutory groups responsible for health promotion among gay men. Examining this approach to HIV prevention in and around London is of particular importance since the prevalence of HIV infection among gay men in the capital is higher than elsewhere in the UK (PHLS 1998).

In the US studies, the men using bars in one city rarely, if ever, went to bars in any other city. The cities were chosen because they were 'discrete, compact' environments. The discrete nature of the gay populations in the cities lent itself admirably to an evaluation where one group of bars received the intervention while others served as controls. While it would be desirable to evaluate an equivalent intervention in gay bars in London, this would be problematic because of population mobility. That is to say, people go to more than one bar. It would be difficult, therefore, to create distinct intervention and control groups using venues where the patrons go from one bar to another, especially in central London (this phenomenon is known as 'contamination' between intervention and control groups). Nor would it be appropriate to use bars in other cities as controls for an intervention introduced in London bars. Epidemiological data clearly indicate that the prevalence of HIV, hence the risk of exposure, is greater among gay men in London than elsewhere in the UK (PHLS 1998). Consequently, gay men living outside London could not serve as suitable controls for people living in the capital.

Thus, although an intervention using peer educators as agents of behaviour change *may* work in gay bars in London, the fluid nature of the customers in London bars argues against formally evaluating the intervention in bars in the capital by means of a controlled trial. For this reason we decided to evaluate a peer-led intervention among gay men who used one of four gyms in central London.

HIV prevention using peer educators in central London gyms

Within central London, four gyms were identified with a large gay membership. Because people usually take out a six- to twelve-month subscription, they tend to go regularly to one gym only. (This was subsequently confirmed during data collection; 92 per cent of the men said they had used only one of the targeted gyms during the study period.) Thus these four gyms with a large gay membership provided the 'discrete, compact' environments required for evaluating a health promotion intervention by means of a controlled trial. A peer-led intervention could be introduced into some gyms while others remained as controls.

To the best of our knowledge, no peer-led programmes have ever been initiated among gay men attending gyms. Methodologically, a gym-based study has some advantages over a bar-based approach for developing and evaluating an intervention. Gym membership is relatively stable over time; people go to the gym regularly; men may spend one to two hours at the gym each time they go, making potential contact with a peer educator feasible; alcohol is not consumed on the premises. The managers of the four gyms responded enthusiastically when we approached them with this project proposal and subsequently gave full support to health promotion and HIV prevention work on their premises. They agreed that within the gyms social networks were quite well defined and peer educators could, in principle, be identified.

Sex and steroids

Going to a gym is an increasingly popular form of recreation in the

UK, and gay men are no exception to this trend. A gym-based intervention could access sexually active gay men, predominantly aged twenty-five to thirty-nine years who are likely to be 'out on the scene'. They represent a notable population at risk for sexually acquired HIV infection. In addition a gym-based study provides the opportunity to examine *steroid use* and injecting behaviour (of steroids) among gay men. Anecdotal evidence suggests that steroid use is increasing among gay men, although there has been no systematic investigation of this. A national survey of steroid use among gym attenders found that the majority of users inject (Korkia and Stimson 1997). Until now, no information has been available on the injecting behaviour of gay men using steroids, and in particular whether they share needles, syringes or multi-dose vials. Were they to do so, this would present an additional risk for HIV transmission.

Thus, a peer-led intervention among gay men in central London gyms could focus on sexual risk behaviour as well as steroid-related injecting behaviour. The aims of this project were: first, to develop a peer-led intervention in central London gyms for reducing the risk of HIV transmission among gay men; and, second, to evaluate the intervention by means of a controlled trial. In the sections that follow, we describe the methodology that was developed for both the intervention and the evaluation.

The intervention

The intervention was managed by the Gay Men's HIV Prevention Team, Camden and Islington Community Health Services NHS Trust, London.

Recruitment of peer educators

Gym managers were asked to identify potential peer educators, according to agreed selection criteria, by observing people using their gym over several weeks. The people selected, regardless of gender or sexuality, were to be popular, well-known, good communicators and belong to a clique or group (i.e. a social network). The potential peer educators were then approached by either the manager or a member of the project team who talked to them about the intervention and asked if they were interested in participating. If interested, they were offered further information and a selection of dates for training.

Training

Training was provided by two members of the Gay Men's HIV Prevention Team, Camden and Islington Community Health Services NHS Trust. It comprised a one-day session (a Saturday from 10.00am–5.00pm) at a central London venue that was convenient for the peer educators. If at all possible the training was held at the gym itself. The range of topics covered and training methods used during the training day are summarised in Figure 11.2.

All the activities were participatory and designed to build on the skills the peer educators already had. Communication skills played a large part in the training, with activities throughout the day to encourage the peer educators to listen, reflect, summarise and impart knowledge. Emphasis was placed on the fact that the peer educators were chosen because they already appeared to have the ability to communicate with others.

The training also addressed the roles and responsibilities of the

---

Figure 11.2   Intervention

Training programme for the peer educators covered:
* HIV infection
  basic facts
  misconceptions

* steroids
  use
  misuse
  safer injecting practice

* new treatments for HIV
* post-exposure prophylaxis
* cross-infection with HIV
* strategies for risk reduction
* referrals to other agencies (e.g. Terrence Higgins Trust)

Training methods include:
* group discussion
* role play
* confidence building

---

peer educators, confidentiality within the gym, implications of being in a position of power, plus trust and personal relationships with gym members.

Peer education in practice

Once trained the peer educators were asked to have at least twenty conversations over the following five months with gay men who used the gym about safer sex, sex within relationships, new therapies for HIV, and steroid use. They were given a T-shirt with the project logo (Figure 11.3), to wear when they were on 'duty', so that they could be recognised as a 'project rep' (the term we used for the peer educators). In addition, sticky labels with the project logo were kept at the gym reception desk. Peer educators could stick one of these labels on a regular T-shirt when they wanted to be 'on duty'. If they wished to work out and not be disturbed they would not wear their T-shirt or a sticker on that occasion.

Support for the peer educators

Peer educators were offered support for their work in a number of ways:

*   Folders were kept at each gym reception which contained additional information (including where to refer people) and leaflets

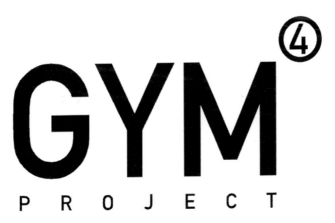

Figure 11.3   The 4 gym project logo

- All peer educators were given the telephone number of the Gay Men's HIV Prevention Team (Health Promotion Services, Camden and Islington Community Health Services NHS Trust) whom they could contact for assistance
- Members of the Gay Men's Team arranged 'surgeries' to meet reps at the gym if requested to do so
- The project team organised a promotion (with posters and leaflets) at the gym at the beginning of the intervention to raise the profile of the project and the role of the peer educators
- An informal social event was arranged for the peer educators and project team members at a central London bar
- A 4 gym project guide was produced with information about the project, hints on how to talk to people, how to deal with different situations and sample questions
- Monthly feedback meetings were held at each gym providing reps with the opportunity to raise issues while the intervention was running.

Peer educators were encouraged to contact the team if they had any queries. Focus groups and feedback sessions were arranged at the end of the intervention when peer educators were asked to make recommendations for improvements and change. (Further details about the intervention are available from Mark Maguire, Health Promotion Service, Camden and Islington Community Services (NHS) Trust.)

Timetable – 'top up'

In three gyms the intervention was introduced once only over a period of several months. In one of the gyms, however, the intervention was introduced at the beginning of the project, then reintroduced twelve months later to see whether a 'top up' had any additional effect. The US studies did not consider whether a top up or 're-inoculation' had any further benefit.

The evaluation

The evaluation was undertaken by the HIV Prevention Unit, Department of Primary Care and Population Sciences, Royal Free and University College Medical School, University College London.

Controlled trial

The intervention was evaluated by means of a controlled trial. The four gyms selected for the project provided 'discrete, compact' environments where the intervention could be introduced at different times – allowing gyms to have intervention and control phases. Once we had set up the study, we were offered access to a fifth gym. Since we did not have the resources to introduce the intervention into the fifth gym, we agreed that gym 5 would serve as a control throughout the study. The name '4 gym project' had already gained a foothold by that time, and so wasn't changed despite the addition of a fifth gym. We understand that of the sizeable gyms in central London, these five attract the largest number of gay men. One gym is exclusively gay; the other four estimate that gay men comprise between 40 per cent to 90 per cent of their male membership (Table 11.1)

The project had three six-month phases (see Table 11.2).

- *Phase 1* – the intervention was introduced into gyms 1 and 2; gyms 3, 4 and 5 served as controls.
- *Phase 2* – active peer education ceased in gyms 1 and 2 (follow-up); the intervention was introduced into gym 3; gyms 4 and 5 remained controls.
- *Phase 3* – the intervention was reintroduced into gym 1 ('top up') and introduced for the first time into gym 4; there was no active peer education in gyms 2 and 3 (follow-up); gym 5 remained a control.

Of the four gyms, two did not express any preference as to when the intervention was introduced, while two did. They asked for the intervention to be introduced during phases 2 or 3 rather than during phase 1. Consequently, randomisation of gyms was not possible. During phase 1, the intervention had to be introduced into the two gyms without a preference (referred to as 1 and 2) while the other two, with a preference (3 and 4) served as controls. The preference for the intervention to be introduced in phases 2 or 3 was solely administrative, was unrelated to the characteristics of the gym membership and should not be a source of bias. Baseline data collected in all gyms allowed us to examine the comparability of the study population in each gym.

Table 11.1 Baseline survey: number of questionnaires distributed and returned

Gym	Number of questionnaires distributed			Number of questionnaires returned			Response rate[4] (%)		
	Overall[1]	to gay men[2]	to straight men[2]	Overall	by gay men[3]	by straight men[3]	Overall	gay men	straight men
1	799	719	80	362	335	27	45.3	46.6	33.8
2	703	280	423	213	137	76	30.3	48.9	18.0
3	1,146	573	573	411	292	119	35.9	51.0	20.8
4	230	230	–	125	125	–	54.3	54.3	–
5	383	191	192	145	115	30	37.9	60.2	15.6
Total	3,261	1,993	1,268	1,256	1,004	252	38.5	50.4	19.9

Notes:
[1]Some men may have taken a questionnaire, mislaid it, and then asked for another which they then completed. Consequently, the number of questionnaires distributed is slightly greater than the number of men to whom they were given.
[2]Managers were asked to estimate what proportion of their male membership was gay. Estimates were: gym 1, 90%; gym 2, 40%; gym 3, 50%; gym 4, 100%; gym 5, 50%. These percentages were applied to the overall number of questionnaires distributed in each gym to obtain the estimated number of questionnaires given to gay and straight men.
[3]According to sexual orientation as reported on questionnaire.
[4]True response rates may be slightly higher, since the denominator (number of questionnaires distributed) may exceed the actual number of men who received them.

Table 11.2 Timetable for the intervention and its evaluation

Month	0	1–5	6	7–11	12	13–17	18
		Phase 1		Phase 2		Phase 3	
Gym 1	Baseline survey Train peer educators	Intervention Peer educators endorse safer sex	Follow-up survey 1	Follow-up No active peer education	Follow-up survey 2 Retrain peer educators	Intervention (top up) Peer educators endorse safer sex	Follow-up survey 3
Gym 2	Baseline survey Train peer educators	Intervention Peer educators endorse safer sex	Follow-up survey 1	Follow-up No active peer education	Follow-up survey 2	Follow-up No active peer education	Follow-up survey 3
Gym 3	Baseline survey	Control	Follow-up survey 1 Train peer educators	Intervention Peer educators endorse safer sex	Follow-up survey 2	Follow-up No active peer education	Follow-up survey 3
Gym 4	Baseline survey	Control	Follow-up survey 1	Control	Follow-up survey 2 Train peer educators	Intervention Peer educators endorse safer sex	Follow-up survey 3
Gym 5	Baseline survey	Control	Follow-up survey 1	Control	Follow-up survey 2	Control	Follow-up survey 3

Outcome evaluation

An anonymous, confidential self-administered questionnaire (available from the authors on request) was developed that included questions on sexual risk behaviour, sexual norms, steroid use and injecting behaviour, psycho-social variables, demographic characteristics plus a glossary of words and phrases in French, Italian, Portuguese and Spanish. The questionnaire was piloted among men using gyms other than the five in the study to determine its acceptability and feasibility.

Primary outcome measures concerned injecting and sexual risk behaviour, including:

- unprotected anal intercourse (UAI) in previous three months
- unprotected anal intercourse in previous three months with a person of unknown or discordant HIV status
- percentage of men ever tested for HIV
- needle-sharing for injecting steroids in previous three months.

Secondary outcome measures are sexual norms and other steroid related risk behaviours including:

- peer group values for safer sex
- personal values about new therapies for HIV
- use of steroids in previous six months.

Information on outcome measures was collected by self-administered questionnaires which were distributed in all gyms at baseline, then after six, twelve and eighteen months at the end of each phase (see Table 11.2). At every stage, questionnaires were distributed in each gym all day, every day for one week. This ensured that all regular gym users were asked to complete a questionnaire. Thus the sample should be representative of men using the gyms. The project team, with the aid of sessional workers, co-ordinated the distribution and collection of questionnaires in each gym over a one-week period.

Four of the gyms are mixed – men and women, gay and straight. Since it was neither feasible nor ethical to ask men if they were gay or straight before handing them a questionnaire, *all men* who came to the gym during the survey period were asked to complete a questionnaire. The questionnaire was divided into sections – some questions to be answered by all men, some by gay men only, some by steroid users only. The baseline questionnaire took about fifteen minutes to complete while the follow-up questionnaires were shorter (five minutes) (copies available on request from the authors). Men were able to take the questionnaire away to complete and return later that week. Collection boxes for questionnaires were left in the gyms during the distribution week and for two weeks afterwards. Questionnaires were collected from the boxes regularly. The comparisons in primary outcomes that could be made at the end of each phase are presented in Table 11.3.

The trial was designed so that:

- after six months the short-term impact of the intervention in gyms 1 and 2 could be compared with the three control gyms (3, 4 and 5)
- after twelve months the longer-term impact of the intervention in gyms 1 and 2 and the short-term impact in gym 3 could be compared with the control gyms (4 and 5)
- after eighteen months the effect of a 'top up' in gym 1 could be compared with the gym where there was no top up (gym 2), as well as with the gym where the intervention has been introduced for the first time (gym 4) and the control gym (gym 5).

Process evaluation

Kelly *et al.* (1991, 1992, 1997) demonstrated that peer education was an effective tool for HIV prevention among gay men in small US towns. They did not, however, reflect on the underlying processes of peer education, why and how it works, the importance of individual personality and practical constraints. Nor were they able to consider issues of transferablity, cultural adaptation and whether peer education works outside the USA.

To better understand the underlying processes of a peer-led intervention, data were collected from peer educators, as well as those who selected, trained and supervised them, using focus groups, personal interviews and self-administered questionnaires. In this way we attempted to establish how and why peer education works and whether it may be transferable to other settings. Information was also recorded on recruitment, training, support procedures and costs.

Table 11.3 Evaluation: primary outcomes to be compared at each survey point

Month	0 Baseline survey	1–5 Phase 1	6 Follow-up survey 1	7–11 Phase 2	12 Follow-up survey 2	13–17 Phase 3	18 months Follow-up survey 3
Gym 1	Baseline measures	Intervention	Changes in risk behaviour immediately after the intervention	Follow-up	Longer term changes in risk behaviour (follow-up)	Intervention (top up)	Changes in risk behaviour immediately after the 'top up'
Gym 2	Baseline measures	Intervention	Changes in risk behaviour immediately after the intervention	Follow-up	Longer term changes in risk behaviour (follow-up)	Follow-up	Changes in risk behaviour without 'top up' (control for gym 1)
Gym 3	Baseline measures	Control	Changes in risk behaviour during control phase (control for gyms 1 & 2)	Intervention	Changes in risk behaviour immediately after the intervention	Follow-up	Longer term changes in risk behaviour after the intervention
Gym 4	Baseline measures	Control	Changes in risk behaviour during control phase (control for gyms 1&2)	Control	Changes in risk behaviour during control phase (control for gyms 1,2,3)	Intervention	Changes in risk behaviour immediately after the intervention
Gym 5	Baseline measures	Control	Changes in risk behaviour during control phase (control for gyms 1 & 2)	Control	Changes in risk behaviour during control phase (control for gyms 1,2,3)	Control	Changes in risk behaviour during control phase (control for gyms 1–4)

Process measures included:

- peer recruitment, selection and retention
- personality profile of the peer educators
- peer educator's motives for participating in the project
- feasibility of setting up and sustaining a peer education programme
- costs of setting up and sustaining a peer education programme
- feedback from peer educators on the number, type and content of conversations held with men in their gym.

Baseline survey: September–October 1997

Response rate

The baseline survey was conducted in the gyms in September–October 1997. Overall, 3,261 questionnaires were distributed to men attending the gyms during the survey period. We asked managers in the mixed gyms to estimate, by giving lower and upper limits, what proportion of their male membership was gay. The number of questionnaires handed out to gay men in each mixed gym was derived by multiplying the total number of questionnaires distributed in that gym by the estimated proportion of the male membership that was gay (using the managers' upper limit). In this way we estimated that questionnaires were handed out to 1,993 gay men and 1,268 straight men (Table 11.1).

Overall, 1,256 completed questionnaires were returned. Respondents were asked to indicate their sexual orientation on the questionnaire; 1,004 questionnaires were returned by men who described themselves as gay (or bisexual) and 252 by men who described themselves as straight. Thus, the estimated response rate for gay men was 50.4 per cent (1,004/1993) and for straight men 19.9 per cent (252/1,268) (Table 11.1). This marked differential in response rates was not altogether surprising since most of the questions concerned sexual risk behaviour for HIV among gay rather than straight men.

The response rate of 50.4 per cent for gay men should be seen as a minimum estimate since we may have overestimated the number of gay men who were handed a questionnaire (the denominator) for two reasons. First, we used the managers' upper limit for the proportion of their male membership that was gay, when calculating the number of questionnaires distributed to gay men. The lower limit would have yielded a smaller number of men, thus reducing the size of the denominator. Second, since the research team visited each gym for a week, some men may have taken more than one questionnaire away with them. The number of questionnaires distributed may, therefore, have exceeded the actual number of men who were given one. Adjusting for both these factors raised the estimated response rate among gay men to 55–60 per cent.

An estimated response rate of 50–60 per cent among gay men in the 4 gym project was slightly lower than anticipated. Surveys conducted in gay bars and clubs in London, as part of the Gay Men's Sexual Health Survey, have reported response rates of 75–80 per cent (Dodds *et al.* 1998, Nardone *et al.* 1998). However, the questionnaires distributed in bars and clubs were short and were filled out on the spot, which undoubtedly contributed to the high response rate. The questionnaire for the 4 gym project was considerably longer, taking about fifteen minutes to complete, which may have influenced the level of response. In addition, there was a substantial number of gym members whose first language was not English. They may have found a long questionnaire with a wide range of questions difficult to complete, despite the glossary of terms in French, Italian, Portuguese and Spanish. The question as to whether non-response is a source of bias in the gym survey is discussed below.

The strength of our questionnaire was that we asked detailed questions about risk behaviour, relationships, barriers to condom use, sexual norms, HIV testing, steroid use and injecting behaviour which could not be included in a shorter survey. A further advantage was that men could complete the questionnaire in private, either at the gym or elsewhere, returning it a few days later. This approach was feasible since most men go to the gym several times a week – an approach that may not work in bar-based surveys where attendance may be less regular.

Social and demographic characteristics

Of the 1,004 gay men who returned a baseline questionnaire, the majority were twenty-five to thirty-nine years old (median age thirty-three years), white, employed, university educated and had lived in London for an average of ten years (Table 11.4). Just over half the respondents were currently in a relationship with a man; the median length of relationship was three years. Two-thirds of the men (67.6 per cent; 670/991) said that most of their friends were gay, a third said some were (32 per cent; 317/991) and only four (0.4 per cent) said that none were. On average men went to the gym three times a week. A quarter of the men had never had an HIV test, just over a quarter had been tested in the previous twelve months while the remainder reported having a test more than a year before the survey. Most men had returned for their test result (97.4 per cent; 711/730) and told someone else about it (93.3 per cent; 681/730).

Sexual risk behaviour

Nearly all the men (94.2 per cent) reported having sex with another man in the *previous three months*. A quarter of the sample (25.5 per cent; 256/1,004) reported having unprotected anal intercourse (UAI) with a man in that period. Of the 256 men reporting UAI in the previous three months, 248 could be classified according to type, number and HIV status of partner(s) for UAI (Table 11.5). Among these 248 men, 163 (66 per cent) reported having UAI with their main partner only, eighteen (7 per cent) with a main and casual partner and sixty-seven (27 per cent) with a casual partner only. The majority of men reporting UAI (207, 83 per cent) reported UAI with one partner only.

Of the 248 men reporting UAI, 140 men (56 per cent) did not know their own HIV status, their partner's or both and were classi-fied as having 'status-unknown' UAI. Not surprisingly, status-unknown UAI was more likely to be reported with a casual rather than main partner. Of the 163 men who reported UAI only with a main partner, 44 per cent were status-unknown. By comparison, for those reporting UAI only with casual partners, or with both main and casual partners, over 80 per cent were status-unknown (p<0.001). This proportion did not appear to vary by number of casual partners for UAI (Table 11.5).

Comparison with other studies

Among the 1,004 men who completed a baseline questionnaire in the 4 gym project, a quarter reported unprotected anal intercourse in the *previous three months*. This is comparable with levels of risk behaviour reported in other community surveys in London. Among gay men surveyed in London bars, clubs and GU services in 1995, 1996 and 1997, approximately one-third reported having had unpro-

Table 11.4   Baseline survey: social and demographic characteristics of
the study population

	Number	Percentage
Age (994)		
<20 yr	1	0.1
20–24	40	4.0
25–29	203	20.4
30–34	336	33.8
35–39	230	23.1
40–44	94	9.5
45–49	49	4.9
>50	41	4.1
Median age (years)	33	
Ethnic group (996)		
White	885	88.9
Black	33	3.3
South East Asian	21	2.1
Other	57	5.7
Employment status (998)		
Currently employed	873	87.5
Years of education (995)		
University or equivalent	722	72.6
Up to A level or equivalent	160	16.1
Up to GCSE or equivalent	113	11.3
Median number of years lived in London (983)	10	
Relationship status (993)		
Currently in a relationship with a man	543	54.7
Length of relationship (540)		
Less than 1 year	119	22.0
Median length of relationship (years)	3	
Had an HIV test (1,000)		
Never tested	270	27.0
<3 months ago	104	10.4
4–12 months ago	178	17.8
Over 1 year ago	448	44.8

Note: The number who answered each question is in brackets.

Table 11.5   Baseline survey: men reporting unprotected anal
intercourse in previous three months

	Men reporting unprotected anal intercourse		
Type of partner for unprotected anal intercourse (UAI)	Status–unknown UAI n (row %)	Status–known UAI n (row %)	All UAI n (row 100 %)
Main partner only	71 (44%)	92 (56%)	163
Main and casual partner(s)	15 (83%)	3 (17%)	18
Casual partner(s) only:	54 (81%)	13 (19%)	67
One casual partner	*36 (82%)*	*8 (18%)*	*44*
More than one casual partner	*18 (78%)*	*5 (22%)*	*23*
All men reporting unprotected anal intercourse	140 (56%)	108 (44%)	248*

Note: *248 men provided information on number, type and HIV status of partner(s) for UAI.

tected anal intercourse in the *previous twelve months* (Nardone *et al.*
1997, 1998, Dodds *et al.* 1998). Between 1993 and 1997, in repeat
surveys conducted at the London Gay Pride festival, about one-
third of gay men also reported unprotected anal intercourse in the
previous twelve months (Hickson 1996).

In many respects the one thousand men in the gym study,
surveyed in September–October 1997, had a similar profile to the
two thousand men in the London bar/club survey conducted two
months later (November–December 1997) (Dodds *et al.* 1998). In
both studies the majority of respondents were white (89 per cent),
young males (median age gym thirty-three years, bar/club thirty-one
years). Similar proportions reported having had an HIV test in the
previous twelve months (gym 28 per cent, bar/club 30 per cent) or
to have ever been tested for HIV (gym 73 per cent, bar/club 67 per
cent). Of the men who reported having unprotected anal intercourse, the proportion who said they did not know the HIV status

of their partner was similar in both samples (just over half). In both studies, employment status, ethnicity and education were not associated with the frequency of UAI while young age was. Compared with the bar/club survey, men in the gym study were more likely to have had a university education (73 per cent *v*. 57 per cent) and be currently employed (88 per cent *v*. 81 per cent), but neither of these were associated with UAI.

In any survey non-response is a potential source of bias, since those who complete a questionnaire may differ from those who do not. The estimated response rate for the 4 gym project (50–60 per cent) was not as high as that reported in other community surveys among gay men (Nardone *et al.* 1998, Dodds *et al.* 1998). Has this introduced bias? We can best answer this question by comparing the gym sample with gay men in the 1997 London bar/club survey (Dodds *et al.* 1998) which achieved an 80 per cent response rate. The bar/club sample is considered to comprise a representative group of 'gay-affiliated' men (i.e. gay men with strong ties to the gay community) in London at risk of HIV. As has already been described, the two groups were similar with respect to a wide range of demographic and behavioural variables (age, ethnicity, frequency of UAI, status-unknown UAI, association of UAI with age, ethnicity, employment and education, and patterns of HIV testing). The belief among HIV prevention workers that there was overlap between these two groups (i.e. many of the same men use a gym and go to bars/clubs) is supported by the similarity of the two groups on many key variables. This suggests that the one thousand men in the gym sample comprise an adequate representation of 'gay-affiliated' men at risk of HIV in London.

The baseline data presented here confirm that the study population in the 4 gym project comprises a sexually active group of gay men, with a sizeable minority at risk for HIV infection. Further analyses will consider unprotected sex within a relationship, the impact of new HIV therapies on risk behaviour, as well as steroid use and injecting behaviour. Baseline measures will provide a point of reference for comparison with data collected at six, twelve and eighteen months follow-up, as part of the outcome evaluation.

Conclusion

There is considerable evidence that HIV transmission is continuing among gay men in the UK. Previous surveys conducted in London found that about one-third of men reported unprotected anal intercourse (UAI) in the previous six to twelve months. In the 4 gym project baseline survey (September–October 1997) one-quarter of gay men reported UAI in the previous three months. Of the men reporting UAI, more than half were unaware of their own HIV status, their partner's, or both.

Peer-led interventions have been shown to be effective in the USA in reducing the level of sexual risk behaviour among gay men. If this approach can be shown to be effective in gyms in London, this would go some way to supporting its introduction into other settings such as gay bars and clubs in London and elsewhere in the UK. The population at risk that could potentially be reached is therefore considerable.

In accordance with the recommendations of the systematic review (EPI Centre 1996), the 4 gym project peer-led intervention has been evaluated by means of a controlled trial. Process evaluation, conducted in parallel, will provide insight into how peer education works – the 'why' and the 'how' of peer education. This chapter has detailed the methodology of both the intervention and evaluation. Subsequent papers will describe sexual risk behaviour in relationships, steroid use and injecting behaviour, the impact of the intervention on HIV risk behaviour and the feasibility of setting up a peer-led intervention in this population.

Acknowledgements

We would like to thank the managers, staff and members of the participating gyms; Glen Monks, Andrew Billington and Will Devlin, Camden and Islington Community Health Services (NHS) Trust; Kaz Lack, Pump Clinic at Signpost; Kim Clarke, Lewisham and Guy's Mental Health NHS Trust. The evaluation was funded by a consortium of inner London health authorities.

References

Cochrane Collaboration (1993) *Introductory Brochure*. Oxford: UK Cochrane Centre.

Dodds J, Nardone A, Mercey D. (1998) *Gay Men's Sexual Health Survey 1997*. London: Department of Sexually Transmitted Diseases, University College London Medical School.

EPI Centre (Evaluation of health promotion and social interventions) (1996) *Review of Effectiveness of Health Promotion Interventions for*

Men who Have Sex with Men. London: London University Institute of Education.

Hickson F., Reid D., Davies P., Weatherburn P., Beardsell S., Keogh P. (1996) 'No aggregate change in homosexual HIV risk behaviour among gay men attending the Gay Pride festivals, United Kingdom, 1993–1995'. *AIDS* 10: 771–4.

Kelly J., St Lawrence J., Diaz Y., Stevenson L., Hauth A., Brasfield T., Kalichman S., Smith J., Andrew M. (1991) 'HIV risk behaviour reduction following intervention with key opinion leaders of population: an experimental analysis'. *American Journal of Public Health* 81: 168–71.

Kelly J., St Lawrence J., Stevenson L., Hauth A., Kalichman S., Diaz Y., Brasfield T., Koob J., Morgan M. (1992) 'Community AIDS/HIV risk reduction: the effects of endorsement by popular people in three cities'. *American Journal of Public Health* 82: 1,483–9.

Kelly J., Murphy D., Sikkema K., McAuliffe T., Roffman R., Solomon L., Winett R., Kalichman S. and the Community HIV Prevention Research Collaborative (1997) 'Randomized, controlled, community-level HIV-prevention intervention for sexual-risk behaviour among homosexual men in US cities'. *Lancet* 350: 1,500–5.

Korkia P., Stimson G. (1997) 'Indications of prevalence, practice and effects of anabolic steroid use in Great Britain'. *International Journal of Sports Medicine* 18: 557–62.

Nardone A., Mercey D., Johnson A. (1997) 'Surveillance of sexual behaviour among homosexual men in a central London health authority'. *Genitourinary Medicine* 73: 198–202.

Nardone A., Dodds J., Mercey D., Johnson A. (1998) 'Active surveillance of sexual behaviour among homosexual men in London'. *Communicable Disease and Public Health* 1: 197–201.

Norton J., Elford J., Sherr L., Miller R., Johnson M. (1997) 'Repeat HIV testers at a London same day testing clinic'. *AIDS* 11: 773–81.

Nutbeam D. (1998) 'Evaluating health promotion – progress, problems and solutions'. *Health Promotion International* 13: 27–44.

Public Health Laboratory Service (PHLS) *AIDS Centre and Scottish Centre for Infection and Environmental Health. AIDS/HIV Quarterly Surveillance Tables.* UK data to end September 1998. 98/3 No. 41

Rogers, E. (1983) *Diffusion of Innovations*. New York: Free Press.

Chapter 12

Falling on deaf ears?

Responses to health education messages from the Birmingham Untreated Heavy Drinkers Cohort

Cicely Kerr, Jenny Maslin, Jim Orford,
Sue Dalton, Maria Ferrins-Brown and
Elizabeth Hartney

Introduction

Over the past three decades there has been a dawning realisation that changes in aspects of individuals' lifestyle can significantly influence their health and longevity and prevent the onset of chronic disease. During this time health education efforts have aimed to bring about positive changes in individuals' health behaviour by communicating information about risks of continuing unhealthy lifestyles and the benefits of adopting a healthier lifestyle. 'Health education attempts to close the gap between what is known about optimum health practice and what is actually practiced' Griffiths (1972: 12). Targets specified in the previous Government's *Health of the Nation* white paper (Department of Health 1992) emphasised the significance of such lifestyle practices. The current Government's consultation paper *Our Healthier Nation* (Department of Health 1998) proposes local Healthy Living Centres specifically aimed at raising local awareness of healthy lifestyle practices.

A common underlying assumption in planning health education efforts is that people adopt risky or unhealthy behaviours because they do not fully understand the consequences of such acts and just do not know any better. Therefore, ignorance is the problem and information the solution. However, although information is necessary, it appears it is not sufficient in itself in creating meaningful change (Wallack 1990) and, despite the efforts of health educators, many individuals continue to engage in behaviours that are known to lead to premature disability and death (Yankauer 1988).

Clearly a greater understanding of these individuals is needed before health educators can hope to influence their behaviour. Campaign planners must know their target audience: the salience of the issue to them, their involvement in it, and where they are cognitively, affectively and behaviourally (Flay and Cook 1981). The consensus of opinion in health education literature is that there is a general need for more formative research informing campaign design (Flay and Burton 1990). Formative research is the primary tool for tailoring public communication efforts to specific audiences, aiming to assess existing knowledge and attitudes of the target population to guide message design.

The consultation paper *Our Healthier Nation* considers the excessive consumption of alcohol as a significant contributing factor in many accidents, domestic violence and poor mental and physical health. By interviewing a sample of 500 individuals drinking at levels likely to cause themselves harm (The Royal College of Psychiatrists 1979), the Birmingham Untreated Heavy Drinkers Project has identified and gathered in-depth information from an important sample of the target audience for alcohol education efforts. As all of these individuals are by definition drinking at unhealthy levels, they are a group which might benefit from lifestyle change and on which existing alcohol education efforts are unlikely to have had sufficient impact. Importantly, all participants had not been treated for their drinking in the last ten years, thus minimising the possibility that contact with clinical services may have influenced their attitudes, beliefs and behaviours.

The aim of this chapter is to explore how respondents maintain their levels of consumption in the face of health information informing them of health risks associated with excessive drinking. As this requires gaining an understanding of the existing knowledge and attitudes of the sample it is important that analysis should be data driven. The issue of alcohol health education was approached qualitatively with the participants in this study by means of open-ended discussion, consistent with an alternative world view in health education put forward by Glanz *et al.* (1990) which relies more heavily on inductive as opposed to deductive methods. However, mindful of their discussion of the danger of ignoring what is known in favour of unstructured research, the findings of this chapter will be discussed with reference to existing theories of health behaviour.

Procedure

Interviews

Respondents were assessed for their fit with the study criteria, namely a consumption of above 35/50 units of alcohol per week (women/men respectively) for at least twenty-seven weeks in the last twelve months, aged between twenty-five and fifty-five years, living or working in the West Midlands conurbation, and having experienced no alcohol-focused treatment in the last ten years. Participants meeting these criteria were invited to attend a two-hour, one-to-one, confidential interview, the time and location adapted to their convenience.

Interviews were carried out by five interviewers trained in both interviewing skills and the collection of data using the partly computerised interview schedule designed for this project (for a copy of the interview manual please contact the authors). The topic of health education was one of a number of areas explored qualitatively during the interview. Information was gathered through open-ended discussion and semi-structured interviewing. All discussions were audio-taped and summarised by means of a comprehensive report written by the interviewer shortly after each interview.

Data collection and qualitative analysis

It is recommended practice in qualitative research to use an iterative procedure whereby analysis commences shortly after the first data are collected, so that later stages of data collection can be informed by earlier stages of analysis (Strauss and Corbin 1990). Thus in the Birmingham Untreated Heavy Drinkers Project, the qualitative data collection and analysis was structured as a three-stage process incorporating progressive refining of the questions asked at each stage. Preliminary analysis took place between stages one and two, and again between stages two and three.

The research data for analysis consisted of transcripts of audio-taped health education focused discussions, the audio-taped discussions themselves, and summaries of the focused discussions detailed in the post-interview reports. Grounded theory analysis of the data was carried out following the guidelines laid down by Strauss and Corbin (1990). Transcripts and post-interview report data were analysed line by line and annotated with words or short phrases encapsulating the meaning. These codes were compared and categorised, conceptually similar data were then grouped together as themes. The content of each data group was used to describe and clarify the properties of the theme under which they were placed. Further examination and comparison of the content of the themes was then carried out to link sub-themes to themes. Group discussions of the findings of the analysis yielded formalised guidelines and questions for the next stage of qualitative exploration.

For the first stage of interviews (n = 12), interviewers were instructed simply to explore the topic of health education with each participant in as open-ended a manner as could be achieved. Analysis of this set of interviews yielded a number of general themes of discussion. This very unstructured and open style allowed the participants to set the agenda themselves. Hence, the structure for the interviews conducted in stage two was based solely on information originating from earlier participants.

The aim at the second stage of interviewing (n = 30) was to initiate a more detailed discussion of aspects of the topic of health education. The interviewers tried to get 'the whole story' for each individual. The analysis conducted after the second stage of interviewing was therefore based on much richer and more widespread data. As a result it was possible to note implied connections between themes and also identify previously indistinct sub-themes. The interview structure for the third stage was focused on making explicit the connections between the themes, clarifying ambiguous areas and ensuring that there was enough depth to the data to enable definitions of distinctive themes and sub-themes.

After the final stage of interviewing (n = 20), there had been sufficient exploration of the topic area to allow important and established themes, along with their interconnections, to be distinguished from unsubstantiated themes, subsequently discarded. The enduring themes were operationalised into a model of how participants in the studied sub-sample appeared to have internalised and acted on alcohol health messages.

The following example shows how one particular theme progressed through the process of further exploration and refined questioning at each stage. In the first stage of interviews, as part of general discussions about health education messages, some participants commented on the source of the messages, intimating that this may have had some impact on their assessment of the value of those messages. As a result of this finding, interviewers questioned second stage participants about where they had gathered their information and awareness of alcohol health matters. Analysis of the second stage interviews revealed a whole host of sources of information and some indication of the effect that particular sources had on an individual's acceptance of the message.

For the final stage of interviewing, the source of health information was highlighted as an area for specific exploration. Interviewers asked participants about who, or what, had given them the most information on the health effects of alcohol, how much they thought the source of the message had affected their belief of that message, and who they felt they specifically would, or would not, listen to about such health matters.

Sample

All participants either lived or worked in the West Midlands Metropolitan County Area (population 2,453,000, 1991 Census figures). In order to reach a varied and representative sample of untreated heavy drinkers, a wide range of recruitment strategies were employed. The project advertised for 'drinkers aged twenty-five to fifty-five to take part in some serious research', in local newspapers, local shops, off-licenses and on buses. Leaflets and free-post postcards were handed out to members of the community in pubs, off-licenses, fairs, markets and car-boot sales. Posters were placed in a wide range of venues including pubs, shops, dental surgeries and work sites. Letters were delivered door to door, and researchers carried business cards with the details of the project on for easy distribution during recruitment and/or work activities. The most successful methods of recruitment were 'snowballing' (word of mouth), where participants who had already taken part told others about the project, and bus advertisements. Both were effective in recruiting hard-to-reach groups such as women, people from ethnic minority groups and those from professional and managerial occupational groups.

The health education focus sub-sample was made up of sixty-two individuals. In the early stages of interviewing, participants were interviewed in the order that they presented themselves to the research project, regardless of their demographic characteristics. However, it was important that as far as possible the health education focus sub-sample would reflect the sample structure of the main sample of 500. Consequently, at the third stage of focused interviewing, participants were selected on the basis of age, gender, employment status, ethnicity and socio-economic grouping (defined using the guidelines of the

OPCS 1980). The aims in terms of sample structure were a balance of male:female in the ratio 3:1 and a representation of the proportions of age, employment status and ethnicity of drinkers modelled on the findings of the 1991 Census for the West Midlands, as well as a balanced representation of socio-economic groups. The characteristics of this sub-sample are shown in Table 12.1.

The sub-sample of sixty-two was made up of forty-five males and seventeen females. The males' ages ranged from twenty-five to fifty-four years, with a mean age of 38.2 years, and their consumption of alcohol over the week prior to interview ranged from 0 to

Table 12.1   Characteristics of the health education focus sub-sample

		Males (n = 45)	Females (n = 17)
Age	25–34	18	8
	35–44	15	5
	45–55	12	4
Activity	Employed	27	8
	Unemployed	13	4
	Unavailable for work	3	3
	Student	2	1
	Housewife/husband	–	1
Socio-economic group	Professional	3	–
	Managerial/technical	6	4
	Skilled non-manual	6	7
	Skilled manual	13	–
	Partly skilled	8	2
	Unskilled	4	1
	Inactive	5	3
Ethnic group	White	42	15
	Black	1	1
	Asian	1	–
	Other	1	1

210 units, with a mean consumption of 93.7 units. For the females, ages ranged from 25 to 48, mean 35.9 years; consumption ranged from 22 to 116, mean 52.2 units of alcohol in the preceding week.

Results

The key themes that emerged during analysis can be grouped under the headings of external influences, internal knowledge, internal barrier and behaviours. The following text describes the content of those themes, illustrative quotes are referenced to the relevant participant (P) number.

External influences

Sources of information

Participants gathered information about health education from numerous sources; most frequently cited were the media, mainly television news and documentaries and newspaper articles. Some individuals had access to more specialist material because they were on a relevant course or they worked in the pub trade. Another common source of information was experience, their own and other people's, passed on through conversations. The consensus of opinion was that some sources of information are definitely more credible than others. The majority of participants felt that GPs are very credible sources, although the following participant, like others, felt strongly that doctors were in no position to give information:

> if the Doctor comes in the room you know giving all this advice … he hasn't been there himself … he doesn't realise what it's like … he hasn't the right to say … unless he's been there himself.
> (P737, male, age forty-one years, consumed 138 units of alcohol in the preceding week)

This participant, like many in the sample, was in favour of the other source thought to be credible, drinkers themselves. Their experience of the issue seemed to be important for credibility.

Medical assistance

Participants showed a strong reliance on their GPs in this area. If they felt ill and thought it might be connected with their drinking, confirmation by their doctor that symptoms were definitely caused by drinking seemed to be a vital piece of evidence of alcohol harm needed before their drinking would be changed.

> You can't just say to somebody, oh it might damage your liver, or it will damage your liver, you need to know your liver is damaged don't you, to make you cut down in anything.
>
> (P205, female, age twenty-eight years, consumed 61 units of alcohol in the preceding week)

Other drinkers

Many of the participants knew other drinkers who had either become ill or died through their drinking, and in these cases they identified the differences between their own and the other's drinking to reassure themselves that their own drinking was not as harmful. They drank spirits when the participant only drank beer, they took drugs as well, they regularly drank in the morning and so on. This process appeared to reassure participants of their own safety despite some being aware that it was a false sense of security:

> kidding myself that I do it openly and he did [it] in secret as though there was some kind of difference.
>
> (P706, male, age forty-eight years, consumed 105 units of alcohol in the preceding week)

Several participants described individuals they knew who had lived unhealthy lifestyles, including substantial drinking, yet had not been troubled by illness and had led long lives. Some took this to mean that in general alcohol is not as damaging across the board as it is made out to be and others relied on the possibility that they might be one of these exceptions who can drink with impunity:

> because I suppose that we all think we're that one tenth that [it] doesn't happen to.
>
> (P722, female, age forty years, consumed 51 units of alcohol in the preceding week)

Similarly, others gained security from the fact that their drinking was similar to those around them, an average level, and that their similar drinking companions were not ill.

Internal knowledge

Awareness

Individuals varied in their level of current awareness both of health risks and recommended limits. The most common awareness level is summed up by P205 (female, age twenty-eight years, consumed 61 units of alcohol in the preceding week).

> I don't know much, not on that … I know it could be bad for your liver, because your liver doesn't renew itself, that's all I know.

Most were aware of some of the health risks particularly liver damage, but it was rare for participants to know how damage occurs or what would be the detectable signs that alcohol had damaged their own health.

Many participants felt that their awareness of the risks of drinking was currently useful to them in limiting their drinking and the recommended levels were helpful as a benchmark against which to compare their own drinking. However participants did not seem to feel any compulsion to stick strictly to the limits.

> I mean I would never be worried in going a bit over the … limits in any way.
> (P044, female, age forty-four years, consumed 116.5 units of alcohol in the preceding week)

Many participants saw awareness in a positive light and wanted to know more, specifically more facts about health effects apart from liver failure and particularly what hangovers meant in health terms. However others felt they knew enough already and the rest was down to them. They did not want to know any more and even felt that an increase in awareness may make their drinking worse because they would have to drink to handle the anxiety it would cause them.

Damage

The majority of the participants were not experiencing any signs of drink-related damage to their health, although many mentioned hangovers in terms of temporary harm unconnected to permanent bodily damage.

> my health deteriorates the next day … when I've got a hangover and a raging headache and I can't sort of productively do anything … but it always goes, you know by the end of the day. So the following day … I don't think it's … had an adverse effect on my health.
>
> (P796, female, age twenty-nine years, consumed 26.5 units of alcohol in the preceding week, less than in a typical week)

A few participants were noting quite specific symptoms, including backache, stomach pains and gout.

Image of alcohol

In this sub-sample, the participants' image of alcohol varied across individuals, with some judging it harshly as a deadly substance and others seeing it in a more positive light as a natural substance better to use than chemicals. In comparison with other substances, many saw it as much less damaging or anti-social than smoking and less harmful, more acceptable and more controllable than drugs. Some individuals did accept that they were less open to messages discouraging drinking than they were to other unhealthy behaviours because it is something they enjoyed so much. They liked to keep it as an area of their life free from restrictions compared to other areas of their life which they feel are already constrained.

Beliefs about aging

Age and aging was a common theme of discussion. Many participants subscribed to the view that an increased awareness of health risks became much more important due the notion, that as you got older, your body could not take drink as it used to. It becomes more important to prolong your life:

> I think it gets worse when you're older … because if you've got a younger body, it's not going to damage as much so I think I'm alright now. I'll carry on for a bit more.
>
> (P715, male, aged twenty-nine years, consumed 51 units in the preceding week)

Participants felt you should moderate your drinking as you got older or expected that a moderation of their drinking would happen naturally as they got older. Participants commonly stated forty as the age when this moderation should start because that is when they felt the damage began and habits were harder to break.

Internal barrier

Perception of severity

While some could accept that they may have done themselves harm through drinking, their feeling of general health and absence of symptoms led them to believe that they had either escaped harm or that any harm was minor:

> If I thought it was serious enough to consider then I would do it but it isn't … in my eyes, in my own eyes, it isn't that serious.
> (P737, male, age forty-one years, consumed 138 units of alcohol in the preceding week)

Those participants who weren't feeling as good as they used to generally put it down to aging rather than drinking. Individuals noting specific symptoms did not see these aches and pains as signs of serious damage and, while they were not getting progressively worse, they could be viewed as temporary or short-term effects.

Deterrence

A minority of participants felt that knowing all the health risks of drinking would frighten them and more information would be likely to lead to them drinking less as a result. However, even when they recognised definite signs of effects of drinking on their health, most participants did not see the effects as serious and so their drinking remained unaffected. The probability of damage to their health was, for the majority, not deterrent enough to affect their drinking.

On the whole participants did not talk about health concerns as relevant to them, although many found other negative effects of drinking worrying. Mostly worries focused around the possibility of becoming dependent on alcohol:

If a lot of mornings a week ... I had to drink to feel better then I'd worry about ... probably I'd worry about needing the drink at first more that the health.

(P715, male, age twenty-nine years, consumed a lower than average 41 units of alcohol in the preceding week)

Participants also found the possibility that drinking might interfere in their functioning in work and relationships and that they might exhibit anti-social behaviour more worrying. That their appearance might suffer, due to weight gain in particular, was also of concern.

Control

When talking about the area of change of drinking patterns and levels, many participants revealed that they did not feel fully in control of their drinking, which was determined by external factors, such as life stress or social events. Individuals believed that they had no restraint and that they could not stop the drinking in such situations, despite awareness of the risks to their health:

if you're that wound up, or you're that upset, or whatever, it doesn't matter what you know, you are not going to stop drinking, you are going to have that bottle until it's empty.

(P722, female, age forty years, consumed 51 units of alcohol in the preceding week)

Other individuals saw their drinking as moderated by their body rather than themselves and hence self-control is already taken care of. Individuals also seemed to expect that their drinking would naturally change to a healthier level through settling down, having to study hard for exams, and growing older and more responsible. It appeared that these individuals did not see changing their drinking as a conscious active process, rather a passive and external one not requiring thought or action.

Benefits of current drinking level

In discussions of this subject area participants gave an insight into what factors defined their current levels of consumption. Many could see disadvantages to both increasing and decreasing consumption from their current level, showing that they saw their current level positively as a balanced one for their own needs. In the main, participants saw reducing their drinking as having many negative effects on areas other than their health, reduction in social life being the most often cited along with reduced enjoyment. Participants also saw the benefits that drinking brought them in areas of social support and coping, increased confidence and optimism, stress relief, relaxation and a good marital relationship. These were more important to them than the risk of harm to their health.

> I consider the benefits that I gain from having a drink outweigh the risks there are.
> (P402, male, age forty-two years, consumed 50.5 units of alcohol in the preceding week)

Behaviours

Harm-reduction behaviours

Participants showed awareness that certain drinking patterns and behaviours were healthier than others. Virtually all were doing something which, in their eyes, reduced the harm that drinking was doing to them:

> If I'm going to have a drink I might as well drink something that's ... recognised as being fairly healthy. French red wine apparently is and also a drop of scotch is, of course, so I think those two things are beneficial to my health rather than harmful.
> (P507, male, age fifty-three years, consumed 72 units of alcohol in the preceding week)

Some participants avoided drinking spirits, while others attempted to limit consumption by only drinking when out and going out later to limit drinking time. Participants tried to rehydrate themselves and flush out their systems by drinking lots of water and having alcohol-free days after heavy drinking or when hung-over. Although participants found moderation of their drinking hard to achieve, they did perceive drinking in moderation as more healthy than abstinence and bingeing.

Many participants viewed their drinking as part of their lifestyle as a whole and felt that healthy behaviours in some areas of their lifestyle, e.g. good diet and exercise, balanced out other unhealthy behaviours e.g. drinking and smoking. This participant sums up the commonly held belief:

> I think providing you keep your engine running reasonably smoothly you can put some pretty crap petrol there.
>
> (P402, male, age forty-two years, consumed 50.5 units of alcohol in the preceding week)

Barrier model

The themes tabled above and the interconnections between them have been operationalised as a model of individual response to alcohol health education. This will be presented as a main simplified model, of which the four sub-systems will then be presented individually for clarity. The components of the model are shown in italics in the accompanying text.

Figure 12.1 shows a simplified model of a participant's response to alcohol health education, starting from the external influence of *alcohol health messages* through internal processes, leading to

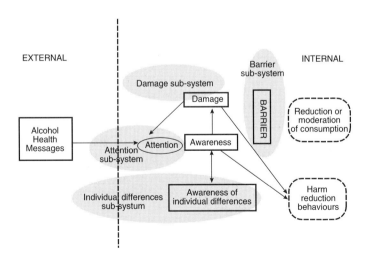

Figure 12.1   Main barrier model

behaviours. The *alcohol health messages* are connected to an individual's level of *awareness* of alcohol health issues through the process of *attention*. The level of *attention* that an individual pays to the *alcohol health messages* is influenced by several internal and external factors, not least the level of *damage* an individual attributes to drinking (see attention and damage sub-systems). An individual's level of awareness in turn affects the attribution of ambiguous health *damage* to alcohol. Linked into the level of *awareness* of alcohol health issues is an *awareness of individual differences* in drinking patterns and effects (see individual differences subsystem). However, the individual's levels of *awareness* and *damage* are barred (see barrier sub-system) from the health educator's desired behavioural outcome of a *reduction or moderation of consumption*. Instead, the individual practices alternative *harm-reduction behaviours*, informed by *awareness of individual differences*.

Figures 12.2–12.5 give details of the influences and processes in the four sub-systems indicated by the shaded areas in Figure 12.1.

Figure 12.2 shows how the *alcohol health messages* enter the internal system through a *source*, which is what the individual attends to. Individual levels of *attention* are affected by the *image of alcohol* that the individual holds, and the individual's *attitude to awareness*, for example whether they feel that an increase in awareness will be useful to them. As mentioned above, the level of *attention* an individual pays to *alcohol health messages* is affected by the level of

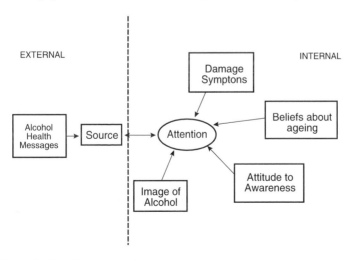

Figure 12.2   Attention sub-system

damage the individual attributes to drinking (see damage sub-system). Additionally *beliefs about aging* influence the age at which participants feel they need to start attending to messages.

Figure 12.3 shows the more complex damage sub-system. Whether an individual connects *symptoms* or health effects to drinking is influenced by level of *awareness* and confused by their *beliefs about aging*. If an individual believes s/he has *symptoms* of *damage* then commonly s/he *seeks medical advice*. If the outcome of *medical help* is that *symptoms* are confirmed as caused by their drinking, the majority of participants maintain that they would *reduce or moderate consumption*. The only other route past the internal *barrier* is a *moderation or reduction of consumption* that participants believe will naturally occur as they get older. Both are speculative routes, however, as no participants in the sample had carried these out. If *medical help* finds *no evidence of damage through drinking*, this serves to maintain part of the *barrier* along with the fact that many participants do not recognise any signs or *symptoms* of *damage* through drinking. As a result of *beliefs about aging*, participants commonly believe damage will not occur until later in life. This, combined with the fact that many participants do not recognise any signs or *symptoms* of *damage* through drinking, contributes to the *perception of the severity* of health risks as low. Consequently health risks do not act as a *deterrent* (see barrier sub-system). Individuals who have signs of *damage* are also in the main not taking the health risks seriously; they practise *harm-reduction behaviours* and do not *reduce or moderate their consumption*.

Figure 12.4 shows another area of processing connected to information individuals gain from *other drinkers*. It appears that individuals note *exceptions and comparisons* to combine with their *awareness* of the health effects of drinking. The resulting *awareness of individual differences* serves to maintain the *barrier* by allowing the individual hope that s/he might be an exception, and the belief that the effects are not as serious as they are portrayed. The same *awareness of individual differences* reinforces and informs *harm-reduction behaviours*.

Finally, Figure 12.5 shows the components of the *barrier* itself and the influences that maintain it. As demonstrated, the above sub-systems maintain the *low perception of severity* and consequently the *low perception of deterrence* of the health risks of excessive drinking. *Low perception of deterrence* is also maintained by other parts of the *barrier* itself: individuals' *low perception of severity* (see damage sub-system); and the *valued benefits of current*

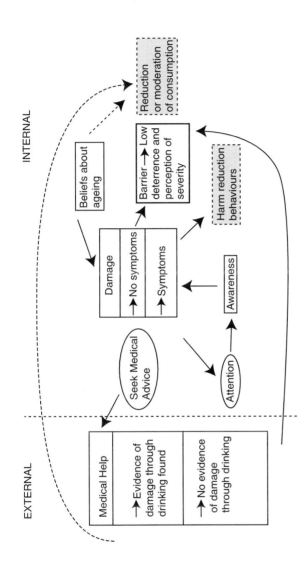

Figure 12.3 Damage sub-system

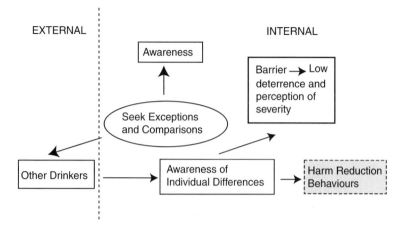

Figure 12.4 Individual differences sub-system

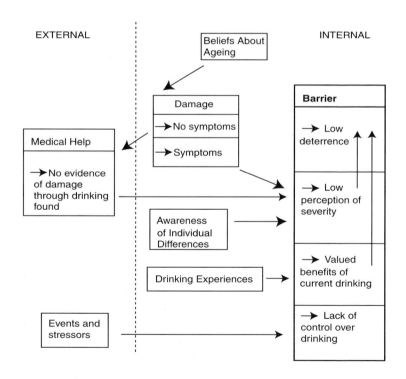

Figure 12.5 Barrier sub-system

drinking. The *valued benefits of current drinking* are based on evaluations of individuals' *drinking experiences* and are important enough to be reason in themselves not to change drinking. The feeling of *lack of control over drinking* is not true of all participants and is not necessarily a constant issue, although the existence of *stressors and events* where individuals feel they would not be able to control their drinking, maintains this part of the *barrier* to change.

Discussion

The complexity of the model and sub-models with all of the influencing themes and interconnections reflects how problematic the route from health education to health behaviour really is. The barrier is made up not just from one stumbling block but four, all of which are actively maintained by people's experiences, thoughts and observations.

It is interesting to note that all four of the components of the barrier correspond strongly to elements which are central to theories of health behaviour, for example the Health Belief Model (Becker 1974). The four major cognitive components of the Health Belief Model (HBM) are, first, perceived susceptibility to a particular health threat; second, perceived severity of the health threat; third, perceived benefits of the behaviour recommended to reduce the threat; and, fourth, perceived barriers to action. 'The combined levels of susceptibility and severity provided the energy or force to act and the perceptions of benefits (less barriers) provided a preferred path of action' (Rosenstock 1974: 332).

In the case of the participants in our study perceived susceptibility and severity are low (severity and deterrence). Participants are able to believe that their drinking is not harmful and will not cause them significant harm. First, this is because they have few symptoms of harm currently, with many possible symptoms being attributed to aging. Second, they dismiss current symptoms of harm as short-term and not severe, referring to acute liver failure as the kind of illness they would consider severe. Third, they feel they have a chance of escaping harm altogether. Weinstein (1982) refers to this as 'unrealistic optimism', finding that people tend to estimate their risk of experiencing a negative event as below average, creating an illusion of comparative invulnerability which will very likely hinder the adoption and maintenance of preventive behaviours.

Additionally in this sample, the costs (perceived barriers) of the preventive action of a moderation of alcohol consumption appear to far outweigh the perceived benefits of the action. Participants seem to have far too much to lose even by dropping their intake of alcohol to more sensible levels.

The other area of the barrier to change is the perceived lack of control over drinking which corresponds with the concept of self efficacy, 'the conviction that one can successfully execute the behaviour required to produce the outcomes' (Bandura 1977: 79). It has been strongly argued that self-efficacy should be incorporated into the HBM, particularly concerning areas involving lifestyle change (e.g. Rosenstock 1990) affecting both the initial adoption of a preventative behaviour and the maintenance of that behaviour over time. Our findings would appear to support this argument.

Awareness does not seem to play as large a role in modifying this apparently risky behaviour as health educators might hope. The majority appears to be aware of the major risk factors and yet they are choosing to continue their excessive drinking. While this may appear disappointing, this is by no means the first time this has been observed. Studies have frequently found that individual ignorance of the main health risks is rare (e.g. Davison 1980), but equally rare is the strong belief that acknowledged 'bad' behaviours, such as smoking or excessive drinking, will always cause illness or death in all those who participate. People do not as a rule believe that behaving in a healthy way will guarantee good health for life.

While this doubt may be frustrating for health professionals, it cannot be seen as purely unfounded. There will always be the cases of the overweight grandfather who drinks and smokes his way to one hundred, and equally the young, fit and healthy man who falls down dead at forty. Lay knowledge is extensive enough that people are aware that health and illness are caused by many factors beyond individual behaviour. Genetic factors, social factors and pure luck are also seen to play a part (Davison *et al.* 1992). Individuals do not see themselves as wholly responsible for, or wholly in control of, their own health. Because of this health educators must be careful to avoid conveying exaggerated claims of predictability and certainty when disseminating information about causality of illness.

It is likely, then, that individuals, such as those in this sample, are continuing to drink at a risky level not through ignorance of the risks, but through an understanding that the risks are not guaranteed to reduce if their drinking is moderated. However, the model suggests that it is not as simple as this either. Individuals have not just thoughtlessly carried on regardless. In many cases they appear to have weighed up the pros and cons of their drinking and through an apparently rational process they have chosen to drink at a particular level. Again this finding is reflected in other research. Graham (1987) found that in the case of cigarette smoking mothers, informants appeared to rationally weigh up the psycho-social benefits of smoking (stress release, inexpensive enjoyment, better performance of roles and responsibilities) against the likely health damage, with the resulting decision to continue smoking.

Participants appear to take a very holistic view of their life and lifestyle in order to make this judgement, with physical health risks being compared with many other areas. It has been suggested that the lay representation of health is not as narrow and unitary as the traditional medical view. In her interviews with French women Herzlich (1973) found three dimensions of health being described. The first was of health as a state of being, an absence of illness. The second was a representation of health as something to be, being able to carry out required and routine roles and responsibilities. In this sample, worries about possible negative effects of drinking focused much more around this aspect of health than physical functioning. The third representation was of health as a state of doing, a positive realisation of an individual's reserve of health, characterised by happiness, relaxation, feeling strong enough to cope and getting on well with others. It is interesting to note how many of the characteristics of this last health dimension were rated as beneficial effects of drinking which would be lost if drinking were to be reduced. Is it possible that, due to differing representations of health, these individuals may feel that they are paradoxically being asked to be less holistically healthy in order to be more physically healthy?

Although participants have given some insight into where they feel health education is lacking in content (how damage occurs, early signs of damage, the health risks signified by hangovers) a more interesting focus of messages could be harm minimisation behaviours. Although participants may not be moderating the quantity of alcohol they consume, they are moderating their drinking pattern or practising healthy behaviours in other areas of their lifestyle in order to minimise the risk of harm to their health through drinking. It would be easy to dismiss many of these behaviours as based on urban myth and hearsay. They are evidence of positively intentioned health behaviour, however, which can apparently be adopted without the costs associated with a moderation of consumption.

There is some promising evidence that health messages are

becoming more compatible with this approach. The emphasis of the most recent campaign of the English Health Education Authority, *Too Much Drink? THINK* (1997) concentrates on behavioural and social consequences of intoxicated behaviour, for example making a fool of yourself socially, making your work suffer. It also gives advice to abstain from drinking for forty-eight hours after a binge to allow the body tissues to recover.

As mentioned at the start of this chapter, a thorough understanding of the thoughts, beliefs and behaviours of the target audience of health education is vital to a successful message. However, it is becoming increasingly clear that, while successfully motivating or persuading people to protect themselves is an important step in disease prevention and health promotion, it is not the whole story. Lay people and professionals alike acknowledge that the responsibility for the nation's health does not and cannot rest solely with the individual. Long-term maintenance of individual-level effects and the ultimate effectiveness of conveying any health messages aimed at effecting lifestyle change must be accompanied by parallel changes in the social environment and social policy in ways that encourage and reinforce the desired changes once individuals make them.

Acknowledgements and disclaimer

This work was commissioned by the Department of Health; the views expressed in this publication are those of the authors and not necessarily those of the Department of Health.

The authors would like to thank everyone involved in the research including the Steering Committee, all those who recruited participants, and particularly the participants themselves. Special thanks also to Sandra Cleaver, Project Secretary, whose particular contribution to so many areas of the project has been invaluable.

References

Bandura A. (1997) 'Self-efficacy: toward a unifying theory of behaviour change'. *Psychological Review* 84: 191–215.

Becker M. (1974) 'The health belief model and personal health behaviour'. *Health Education Monographs* 2: 324–473.

Census County report (1991) West Midlands (part 2). London: HMSO.

Davison C., Frankel S., Davey Smith G. (1992) 'The limits of lifestyle: reassessing "fatalism" in the popular culture of illness prevention'. *Social Science and Medicine* 34: 675–85.

Davison L. (1980) 'An analysis of knowledge, beliefs and behaviour relating to the development of coronary heart disease'. *Health Education Journal* 39: 103–9.

Department of Health (1992) *The Health of the Nation: A Strategy for Health in England.* London: The Stationery Office.

—— (1998) *Our Healthier Nation: A Contract for Health.* London: The Stationery Office.

Flay B., Burton L. (1990) 'Effective mass communication strategies for health campaigns'. In: C. Atkin and L. Wallack (eds) *Mass Communication and Public Health: Complexities and Conflicts.* Newbury Park: Sage, pp. 129–46.

Flay B., Cook D. (1981) 'Evaluation of mass media prevention campaigns'. In: R. Rice and W. Paisley (eds) *Public Communications Campaigns.* Newbury Park: Sage, pp. 175–96.

Graham H. (1987) 'Women's smoking and family health'. *Social Science and Medicine* 25: 47–56.

Griffiths W. (1972) 'Health education definitions, problems, and philosophies'. *Health Education Monographs* 31: 12–14.

Glanz K., Lewis F., Rimer B. (eds) (1990) *Health Behaviour and Health Education.* San Francisco USA: Jossey-Bass.

Health Education Authority (1997) *Too Much Drink? THINK.* London: HEA.

Herzlich C. (1973) *Health and Illness: A Social Psychological Analysis.* London: Academic Press.

Office of Population Censuses and Surveys (OPCS) (1980) *Classification of Occupations.* London: HMSO.

Rosenstock I. (1974) 'Historical origins of the health belief model'. *Health Education Monographs* 2: 328–35.

—— (1990) 'The health belief model: explaining health behaviour through expectancies'. In K. Glanz , F. Lewis, B. Rimer (eds) *Health Behaviour and Health Education.* San Francisco USA: Jossey-Bass, pp. 39–62.

Royal College of Psychiatrists, The (1979) *Alcohol and Alcoholism.* London: Tavistock.

Strauss A. and Corbin J. (1990) *Basics of Qualitative Research: Grounded Theory Procedures and Techniques.* Newbury Park: Sage.

Wallack L. (1990) 'Improving health promotion: media advocacy and social marketing approaches'. In C. Atkin and L. Wallack (eds) *Mass Communication and Public Health: Complexities and Conflicts.* Newbury Park: Sage, pp. 129–46.

Weinstein N. (1982) 'Unrealistic optimism about susceptibility to health problems'. *Journal of Behavioural Medicine* 5: 441–57.

Yankauer A. (1988) 'Disease prevention: still a long way to go'. *American Journal of Public Health* 78: 1,277–8.

Chapter 13

Older people's perceptions about health behaviours over time in Ireland

Implications for health promotion

Anne MacFarlane and Cecily Kelleher

Introduction

The adaptive way in which diverse cultures respond to illness has been examined within the conceptual framework of medical pluralism (Good 1990). Defined as the way in which alternative medical systems 'co-exist and compete with each other within a given culture' (Stainton-Rogers 1991: 21), medical pluralism draws attention to the *diverse* nature of health-related knowledge, attitudes and behaviour. Research of this kind is hugely relevant to health promotion because the motivating forces behind pluralistic practices can be understood and, moreover, the conditions and contexts in which positive and negative health behaviours might occur can be explored.

In Ireland, a innovative national initiative by the Folklore Commission of Ireland in the late 1930s, entitled the Schools' Scheme, resulted in a major archive of traditional medical practices in Ireland. Senior class national school pupils, aged between ten and fourteen years, were invited to become folklore collectors and asked to record material about a range of socio-cultural practices, including traditional folk medicine, from family members and neighbours in essay form. Approximately 50,000 schoolchildren participated and an estimated 20,000 tonnes of written material was gathered (O'Cathain 1988). The collected essays, stored in the Department of Irish Folklore, National University of Ireland, Dublin, contain information about local cures, the use of herbs for healing purposes and visits to Holy Wells.

In 1993/94, the 1930s methodology was replicated in both an urban and rural area to assess the contemporary prevalence of Irish folk medicine, complementary medicine and biomedicine (Murphy

1995), allowing a comparative analysis over time. Some similarities between the 1930s and 1990s database were found. In particular, knowledge about folk remedies and the conditions for which they could be used were remarkably similar. However, differences in practices between the 1930s and 1990s databases were also recorded. A decline in reported utilisation for traditional folk medicine was noted, particularly among participants from non-manual back-grounds (MacFarlane and Kelleher 1997), while knowledge and use of complementary medicine was moderately high (Murphy and Kelleher 1995).

The existence of the two cross-sectional databases described above (O'Cathain 1988, Murphy 1995) was perceived as an oppor-tunity to examine the way in which health-related beliefs and practices might change over time. Therefore, a national interview study with older people in Ireland who, by virtue of their age, may have participated in the 1930s folklore scheme[1] was undertaken. This group of older people were considered interesting not just as older people, but, also, as people who *got older* between the 1930s and 1990s. In this way, ideas about health and illness, behaviours used to maintain and promote health, as well as practices used in response to illnesses, could be examined over time. The purpose of the present chapter is to report on older people's perceptions of health behaviours over time.

Studies of health behaviour aim to attend to self-defined rather than medically defined practices (e.g. Harris and Guten 1979). This is important because the ideas people have about health are not always consistent with 'formal' advice from medical authorities. Qualitative ethnographic work about lay health beliefs in the UK, for instance, has highlighted that public accounts of health and illness reflect 'correct' biomedical views about disease causation. In contrast, private accounts are based on personal experience, social observations and, generally, are more complex and contradict formal health messages (Cornwell 1984, Blaxter and Paterson 1982).

The distinction made by Radley (1994) between health-directed and health-related behaviour is also important in this regard. This means that, while people may be aware of the health consequences of certain activities, health-maintenance or health promotion may not be the primary objective. Indeed, certain activities that may be good for health may be a result of habit, or of other attendant circumstances, and may not be conscious or manifest efforts toward health at all.

Studies about health behaviours have also shown that previous lifestyles are often perceived to be more health-enhancing than contemporary lifestyles. Herzlich's (1973) study in urban and rural France found that life in the past, particularly in rural areas, was perceived to be more healthy than present day life. Similar findings have been reported by Blaxter and Paterson's (1982) UK research and McCluskey's (1989) study in Ireland. Specific health-enhancing features of past lifestyles cited within these studies include references to natural and wholesome food, less stress and stronger people who worked harder. Modern life was considered negative for one's health because of the increased pace of life, unhealthy processed food, pollution, excessive smoking and drinking. Interestingly, when social and economic hardship and ill-health experienced in the past were acknowledged, participants still insisted that they were healthier. Sometimes, it was argued that people benefited or thrived in the face of adversity, particularly from hard work (Blaxter and Paterson 1982). The point that such accounts are rose-coloured representations of the past, resorting to conventional presentations of a 'golden age', has been made strongly (ibid. 1982).

Methods

Participants

The target population for the present study was older people aged between sixty-nine and seventy-two years. Sampling was conducted in collaboration with the National Council for the Elderly and the Economic and Social Research Institute (ESRI), Dublin.[2] Drawing from a 1993 ESRI national probability sample of 909 persons aged sixty-five and over resident in private households, it was calculated that there were 247 people within the relevant age group. These people were invited by letter to complete a short questionnaire on health practices and to participate in an interview, if agreeable. Standard follow-up procedures for postal surveys, as recommended by Miller (1991) were employed. One-hundred-and-twenty-seven replies were received (response rate 51 per cent). Of these 60 per cent (n = 79) expressed an interest in participating in the main inter-view study. Reported utilisation of folk medicine and complementary medicine did not differ significantly between postal survey participants who indicated their availability for the interview study and those who did not. Of the seventy-nine postal survey participants who indicated their availability for the interview study, fifty-one completed interviews (response rate 65 per cent).[3]

A demographic and socio-economic profile of the interview sample was developed from the 1993 ESRI database of those over-sixty-five in Ireland (see Table 13.1). There were no significant differences between participants and non-participants of the interview study apart from the fact that those interviewed had slightly higher levels of formal education (chi square = 15.25 p<0.05).

Design and procedure

The postal survey questionnaire was employed primarily as a means of recruiting participants for the main interview study. The interview study involved the use of a semi-structured questionnaire based on psychological and sociological constructs considered relevant to health beliefs and health behaviours.[4] Participants were asked to discuss their definitions of health, causation theories, health-maintenance behaviours and to identify illnesses experienced by them and/or a family member for three life stages: childhood (0-twenty years), younger adulthood (twenty to forty-five years) and older adulthood (forty-five to present years). As stated earlier, this chapter focuses on reported health behaviours only.

Table 13.1   Demographic and socio-economic profile of interview study participants

		n (%)
Gender	Male	25 (49)
	Female	26 (51)
Marital status	Married	36 (70)
	Widowed/Single	15 (30)
Social class	1	6 (12)
	2	10 (20)
	3	12 (23)
	4	8 (16)
	5	10 (20)
	6	5 (9)

Interviews were conducted in eighteen counties of the Irish Republic between October 1995 and March 1996 within participants' homes and taped with the permission of those being interviewed. On average, interviews were between fifty and sixty minutes in length. All interviews were then transcribed for analysis.

Data analysis

Collected interview data were analysed using content analysis techniques as defined by Holsti (1969) and Krippendorf (1980) using QSR.NUD.IST (Richards and Richards 1994), a software package that helps researchers to manage and explore qualitative data, to link ideas and construct theories about data. Statistical summary reports, e.g. frequency analyses can also be generated.

Criteria for category construction were drawn from Bromley's (1977) work regarding the development of procedural rules and Morse's (1994) description of an audit trail. These criteria were employed to place the creativity and intuition of data analysis in a careful and rigorous context (May 1994) in order to enhance the reliability and validity of the work. The independent rate of agreement for the analysis process was 77 per cent. The final consensus rate of agreement was 96 per cent.

Findings

Beliefs about causes of health and illness, and accounts of practices employed to maintain health and prevent disease, were coded as Determinants of Health. As shown in Table 13.2, there were five sub-categories within the Determinants of Health category with further sub-classifications. Four of these sub-classifications are relevant to the present chapter. These are diet, activity, psychological and social factors.

Diet

Overall, perceptions of childhood dietary patterns were mainly associated with a *lack* of illness and as a means of maintaining health. While a 'poor diet' was cited as a cause of tuberculosis by some participants, most emphasised the fact that they were encouraged to eat 'good food' as children, food that was 'healthy', 'ordinary' and 'wholesome'. It was also made clear by participants

Table 13.2   Reported determinants of health: sub-categories and their sub-classifications

Behavioural	Diet
	Activity
	Smoking
	Alcohol
	Preventive Measures
Psycho-social	Psychological
	Social
	Religion
Environmental	Physical Environment
	Accidents
Biological	Physiological
	Infectious
	Heredity
	Developmental
Other	

that they did not have a lot of choice about food in the past and that 'you ate what was put in front of you and that was it'. The absence of any nutritional advice or guidelines was also noted.

This situation was contrasted with current dietary practices. First, organic production of food in the past was contrasted, mainly by male participants, with the current utilisation of chemicals. Specifically, it was explained that, in the past, no preservatives were used and farming was, therefore, 'what is now termed as organic'. References were made to the increased use of insecticides and growth hormones for animals. Reasons for such changes provided by interviewees tended to emphasise the commercial aspect of farming:

but they (vegetables) were grown naturally (in the past). They weren't forced up, you see. They, how shall I put it, it wasn't the financial garb. They're forcing them out of the ground now. They're not giving them a chance to grow.

The negative effects of changes in food production were described by participants in terms of both health hazards and poor quality food. Specific references were also made to the BSE scare by some participants, although not as many as might have been expected, given the extensive media coverage of the issue in recent times. The reduced quality of food products was discussed in terms of taste. One man described his surprise at the quality and taste of organic vegetables:

> Have you ever tasted the food you get nowadays? I happened to have a recent experience – I bought some organic carrots. They actually tasted like carrots, I couldn't believe it … we buy carrots all the time – they *look* like carrots but they *don't taste* like them. There's something very nasty going on.

Second, perceptions of an increased reliance on processed food, rather than home-grown or home cooked food, were evident. This view was expressed mostly by women and appeared to be implicitly critical of women of the younger generation, specifically participants' daughters and daughters-in-law. Ready-made food, 'packaged' or 'quick' food were dismissed as being inferior to home made food. Negative perceptions of processed food were obvious in the language employed in these data. For instance, one woman stated that she had 'never filled her basket with the kind of *rubbish* you get today' (emphasis added). All the participants emphasised the benefits of home cooking.

General critical comments about contemporary dietary habits were also expressed. It was suggested, for instance, that people ate more 'sweet things' and 'junk food' nowadays and this was sometimes linked with the greater availability of food. One participant was horrified that her grandchildren would have soft drinks with their dinners rather than milk. Similarly, another participant was critical of his grandchildren's eating habits. His views on the matter provide a clear summary of the perceived difference over time regarding dietary patterns:

> I think there is too much sweet things, too much shops, all those Taytos (crisps) and different things. Children go for all those new things that come out. They are all the time eating. My

time, you might get a few sweets once a month when they'd go to town, that was all. There was no such thing as currant cake when we were growing up. You'd have it for Christmas day or maybe the day the turf was being saved, that was about all.

Finally, the absence of any nutritional advice or guidelines in the past was commented on and contrasted with the current level of information people receive about healthy eating. The way in which people managed in the past was emphasised, as was the confusing or contradictory nature of current nutritional advice. Conflicting messages about butter and low-fat spreads were cited as an example of this. Overall, there was a sense of puzzlement, if not annoyance, at the idea of nutritional advice.

Activity

Activity was typically described as health-enhancing by partici-pants. This was particularly evident within reported accounts of childhood health status. Descriptions of active lifestyles during participants' childhood years included references to daily walking and cycling, for example:

> We were never sitting down. I can hardly remember sitting down when I was young. If you had to go anywhere, if you had to go for a message, you either ran it, walked it or cycled it. There were no cars, no tractors, you know. We were very active. We played games nearly every evening and weekends … we were very active.

The increased reliance on cars for transport purposes was discussed in relation to a reduction in physical activity. The practice of driving children to school was singled out by several participants as illustra-tive of an unhealthy feature of contemporary lifestyle. One woman's frustration at this situation is evident below:

> Ninety per cent of the time, they get the car. I mean if they're only going up for a message to the village, it's only a five minute walk, do you think they'd walk? Not at all. I only go up for the pension and the one says to me 'And you walked up? as if I was really doing something extraordinary and it's only one hundred yards up the way.

However, paradoxically, it was also noted that participants did not respond very positively to efforts by people to exercise. One man, from a rural area, remarked on the number of young mothers he saw walking along the road and questioned what was it all for? Another woman explained that, in the past, they did not need to go for long walks or, indeed, that they had no time for that:

> We didn't have to exercise because we got plenty of it with hard work. Nowadays all people think about is going out for long walks, we hadn't time to do that when we were young.

Psychological and social factors

Relatively consistent accounts of hardship and poverty were reported by participants in relation to their childhood years. The broad picture was that unemployment levels were high and money was scarce. References were made to life being 'tough' and 'hard'. The lack of central heating, electricity and sanitation facilities was discussed. One woman provided a detailed description of tenement accommodation in Dublin city during the 1930s:

> The centre of the city was full of tenements in those days and families lived ten to a room – all the children, father and mother. The beds were in one corner, and the table where they cooked was in the other, and the fire, all in one room. Then, they had to go down flights of stairs to the back yard to get water from the tap and go to the toilet outside.

While some references were made to assistance from voluntary or religious organisations, it was generally reported that there was no assistance available for people such as there is today. The extent to which people relied on each other for assistance was discussed at length by several participants.

The tendency to reflect on such difficult social and economic circumstances in a positive light was noted in these data. There seemed to be two notions within this attribution. First, participants would comment on the fact that people *managed* in the face of adversity, or did not experience illness, despite the appalling conditions. For instance, a woman who described previous living conditions in detail completed her discussion with the statement that they had managed and were happy. Similarly, in another interview, as a man recounted the details of living conditions in the past, his wife, who was present, interjected and focused on the fact that people had managed and *survived*. Comments from the participant's wife are shown in brackets:

> Oh, it would be shocking. You'd be trying to live in a very small house you know (small little houses and no ventilation and they had no fresh air). Just across from us here is a little house. This room now isn't as big, and there was five children reared in it (*but they got on all right there*) (emphasis added).

Second, it was found that some participants reported that they were healthy as children *because* of the hardship they experienced then. This view was generally articulated in terms of being hardy. Hardiness was described by some participants in terms of surviving through difficult times, which reflects a physical hardiness. Hardiness as a psychological ability to cope with tough situations and daily struggles was also emphasised.

Comparisons between participants in their youth and the current younger generation were commonly made here also. While people in the past were described as 'hardy', the current generation were considered 'soft', as 'not one bit tough' and also 'lazy'. These differences were attributed to improvements in social and material circumstances in terms of young people being 'spoilt' because they had, for example, the comfort of central heating. Negative lifestyle changes were also mentioned. Social contact and support at community level, enjoyed by people in the past and used as a means of buffering stress, was contrasted with contemporary society. Contact with neighbours were perceived as low and, also, it was said that people were creating stress for themselves because the pace of life was so fast and they were constantly 'chasing' themselves.

Discussion

In this study, older people were asked to discuss the health behaviours of their childhood years. Within these discussions, the impact these behaviours had on health and comparisons between the past and present were made in terms of certain lifestyle behaviours and, also, psychological and social factors. Descriptions of previous and current lifestyles provided by participants in the present study can generally be seen to emphasise the past in positive terms while contemporary lifestyles were regarded more negatively. Representations of the past documented in the present study were rose-coloured in the sense that the way people lived was viewed as predominately health-enhancing. Lifestyle features from the past considered particularly good for health were the levels of activity and work engaged in and the natural, wholesome diet consumed. Aspects of contemporary lifestyles identified as bad for health included the increased pace of life and lower levels of social support at community levels. These findings are consistent with previous retrospective research with older people (e.g. McCluskey 1989, Blaxter and Paterson 1982, Cornwell 1984).

A key question is whether some 'objective' support for these subjective views can be found. An analysis of changes in the food chain since the Great Irish Famine (National Nutrition Surveillance Centre 1995) shows that the mid-1930s diet was relatively low in fat and high in carbohydrates which is better than the current Irish diet which is high in fat and low in carbohydrates. This analysis also showed that while the calorie intake was greater during that period, the calorie output was higher because of daily activities undertaken.

However, notwithstanding this, morbidity and mortality caused by poor socio-economic circumstances of that era cannot be over-looked. Tuberculosis, for instance, was a major public health problem in Ireland through to the 1940s until socio-environmental changes were made to prevent the disease and until appropriate health services were developed for its treatment (Barrington 1987). Indeed, participants did recount stories of family members, neighbours and friends contracting tuberculosis and, in many cases, dying. In addition, life expectancy at birth in Ireland has increased considerably, by eleven years for women and by eight years for men since 1950 (Department of Health 1994). Thus, it seems the overall positive representation of Irish life in the past presented here is selective.

It is argued that a closer analysis of the interviews shows greater acknowledgement of the association between socio-economic factors and health. While childhood diets discussed by participants were described as healthy and 'wholesome' they acknowledged that, in the past, people 'ate what was put in front of them' because 'that was all that was available'. Essentially, there was not much choice. Similarly, while participants described with pride the active nature of their childhood lives and attributed good health status to this, they did explain that this was related to the fact that there were no cars or tractors or buses available. Therefore, again, there was no choice but to be active.

This acknowledgement of the social and economic context of health behaviours was also evident within explanations for lifestyle changes over time. The amount of 'rubbish' eaten by younger people was understood to reflect the fact that people had more money and that there was a wider range of foods available. Similarly, one woman, reflecting on the hardiness of her generation versus the 'softness' of her grandchildren and their peers, commented:

> You see there was no central heating, em, we were hardy really. People nowadays are softer, not one bit tough. I'm not blaming them for that. I think it's just the conditions are generally – the houses now are much more comfortable.

Another force of influence identified within the present analysis relates to social norms as they impact on health-seeking behaviour. The matter-of-fact manner in which participants described the healthy nature of their childhood diet or activity supports the interpretation of these health practices as somewhat unconscious. That is to say that certain lifestyles features, while beneficial for health, were not conscious or formal efforts to maintain or achieve good health. As stated above, such practices were a function of social and economic circumstances, a function of social deprivation and were not borne out of choice. Such practices were just what was normal. This interpretation is consistent with Graham's (1984) analysis of women's roles as carers in which the impact of material conditions and daily routines on behaviour was highlighted. Graham's (1984) conclusions focused on the need for health practitioners and policy-makers to attend to the routines of life which may or may not facilitate health-enhancing practices.

Such analyses are, of course, also consistent with health promotion as outlined in the Ottawa Charter (1986). The Charter urges the development of supportive environments, healthy public policies and community participation, all of which should produce contexts and conditions conducive to health-promoting behaviours and lifestyles.

Interestingly though, the present analysis also revealed a somewhat negative attitude toward health promotion among those interviewed. These must be juxtaposed against participants' negative views of contemporary lifestyles and, specifically, the critical comments made about unhealthy eating and sedentary lifestyles. Why should participants be so vocal and negative about the very issues about which they themselves expressed concerns? An explanation for this may relate to the retrospective nature of participants' attributions of good health to lifestyle practices. The point has been made that these were neither conscious nor chosen practices. In fact, whether the health-enhancing features of these behaviours were recognised at the time is unclear. Participants' accounts of positive health behaviour in the past are, therefore, conceptually consistent with notions of health-related, rather than health-directed, behaviour, as discussed by Radley (1994). Their reactions to health-directed behaviours among younger people were found to reveal a sense of discomfort.

In conclusion, previous evidence of positive representations of past lifestyles by older people, in the UK and France, was further supported by this Irish study. It has been argued that accounts of a healthier lifestyle in the past in terms of diet and activity, in particular, do reflect things as they were but, also, tend to over-emphasise positive features. However, it has also been argued that participants are cognisant of the way in which social and economic factors impact on people's health. For them, certain features of their lives were health-enhancing, but not health-directed. The key issue seems to be that participants, in the past, did not enjoy a sense of choice around their health because of social deprivation but their accounts of that time emphasise what was good for them, rather than what was not. What is also interesting is that their observations of improvements in social circumstances were regarded in negative terms. They discussed the way in which better housing or greater food availability was harmful for health. Moreover, they expressed reticence about efforts to tackle contemporary lifestyle features that are recognised formally as damaging. This might be explained by a cultural shift in society whereby conscious or direct attention to health is acceptable nowadays while it was not in the past. Notwithstanding concerns about the negative aspects of healthism (Skrabanek and McCormack 1990) this shift should be considered positive for health promotion in that thinking about healthy living and aiming consciously to live healthily become socially 'normal'. The key challenge, however, for health policy-makers and those working in health promotion, is to ensure that all people are supported and enabled equally to be conscious of, and about, their health.

Acknowledgements

This research was funded by the National University of Ireland, Galway which provided a postgraduate research fellowship for the first author from 1992–1995 and the Cardiovascular Disease and Health Promotion Research Group (CHIRP), Health Promotion Unit, Department of Health, Dublin. Thanks to members of the Department of Irish Folklore, National University of Ireland, Dublin, the National Council for the Elderly, Dublin and the Economic and Social Research Institute, Dublin for their collaboration and assistance with this work. Thanks to all those who participated in this study for their time and generosity. Finally, thanks to an anonymous reviewer for suggestions and comments.

Notes

1   An exploration of the 1930s archive in the Department of Irish Folklore, University College Dublin was conducted to locate interview study participants' childhood essays. Childhood essays of fourteen interviewees (27 per cent) were traced. This allowed some analysis of individual accounts of non-biomedical practices from two life stages, although it is not within the scope of this article to elaborate.
2   The ESRI undertook a study for the National Council for the Elderly on the health and autonomy of people aged sixty-five years and over in Ireland in 1993 (see Fahey and Murray 1993).
3   Reasons for non-participation were mainly related to the logistics of conducting a national interview study. Data collection comprised seven regional fieldtrips and sometimes participants were not available for interview when the interviewer was in their area. Call backs were not possible because of the distances involved. Also, because the interview study took place during winter months, ill-health prevented participation in a small number of cases.
4   Psychological and sociological constructs employed in the development of the interview schedule include: definitions of health (McCluskey 1989), value of health and locus of control (Wallston *et al.* 1978), health belief model (Rosenstock 1974), illness behaviour (Mechanic 1989) and sickness behaviour (Parsons 1951).

References

Airhihenbuwa C. (1995) *Health and Culture: Beyond the Western Paradigm.* Newbury Park: Sage.
Barrington R. (1987) *Health Medicine and Politics in Ireland 1900–1970.* Dublin: Institute of Public Administration.
Blaxter M., Paterson E. (1982) *Mothers and Daughters: A Three-Generational Study of Health Attributes and Behaviour.* London: Heinemann.

Bromley D. (1977) *Personality Description in Ordinary Language*. London: Wiley and Sons.

Cornwell J. (1984) *Hard Earned Lives: Accounts of Health and Illness from East London*. London: Tavistock.

Department of Health (1994) *Shaping a Healthier Future: A Strategy for Effective Healthcare in the 1990s*. Dublin: Department of Health.

Fahey T., Murray P. (1993) *Health and Autonomy among Over-65s in Ireland*. Dublin: Economic and Social Research Institute.

Good C. (1990) 'Medical pluralism'. In: R. Ornstein, C. Swencionis (eds) *The Healing Brain: A Scientific Reader*. New York: Guilford Press.

Graham H. (1984) *Women, Health and Family*. Falmer, Sussex: Wheatsheaf.

Harris D., Guten S. (1979) 'Health protective behaviour: an exploratory study'. *Journal of Health and Social Behaviour* 20: 17–29.

Herzlich C. (1973) *Health and Illness – A Social Psychological Analysis*. London: Academic Press.

Holsti O. (1969) *Content Analysis for the Social Sciences and Humanities*. Mass. USA: Addison-Welsey.

Krippendorf K. (1980) *Content Analysis: An Introduction to its Methodology*. London: Sage.

MacFarlane A. (in press). 'Concepts of health and illness among older people'. In: C. Kelleher, E. Edmondson (eds) *Health Promotion: Multi-Discipline or New Discipline?* Dublin: Irish Academic Press.

MacFarlane A., Kelleher C. (1997) 'Contemporary health practices in Ireland: manual versus non-manual differences' (letter). *Irish Medical Journal* 90: 240.

MacLachlan M., Carr S. (1994) 'From dissonance to tolerance: toward managing health in tropical countries'. *Psychology and Developing Societies*. 6: 119–29.

May K. (1994) 'Abstract knowing: The case for magic in method'. In: J. Morse (ed.) *Critical Issues in Qualitative Research Methods*. Thousand Oaks: Sage.

McCluskey D. (1989). *Health: People's Beliefs and Practices*. Health Promotion Unit, Department of Health, Dublin: Government Publications Office.

Mechanic D. (1989) *Painful Choices: Research and Essays on Health Care*. New Jersey: Transaction Publishers.

Miller D. (1991) *Handbook of Research Design and Social Measurement* (5th edition). Newbury Park, CA: Sage.

Morse J. (1994) 'Qualitative research: fact or fantasy?' In: J. Morse. (ed.) *Critical Issues in Qualitative Research Methods*. Thousand Oaks: Sage.

Murphy A. (1995) 'Contemporary health practices in Ireland: an urban/rural analysis'. Unpublished MA Thesis, University College Galway.

Murphy A., Kelleher C. (1995) 'Contemporary health practices in the Burren, Co. Clare'. *Irish Journal of Psychology* 16: 38–51.

National Nutrition Surveillance Centre (1995). *Changes in the Food Chain Since the Time of the Great Irish Famine*. Report III. Centre for Health Promotion Studies, NUI: Galway.

O'Cathain S. (1988). *Suil siar ar Sceim na Scol* (*Looking Back over the Schools' Scheme*) 1937/1938. *Sinsear* 5: 19–30.

Ottawa Charter for Health Promotion (1986) *An International Conference on Health Promotion*. Ottawa, Ontario, Canada.

Parsons T. (1951) *The Social System*. Glencoe, Ill: Free Press.

Radley A. (1994) *Making Sense of Illness: The Social Psychology of Health and Disease*. London: Sage.

Richards L., Richards T. (1994) 'From filing cabinet to computer'. In: A. Bryman, R. Burgess (eds) *Analysing Qualitative Data*. London: Routledge.

Rosenstock I. (1974) 'The health belief model and preventive health behaviour'. *Health Education Monographs* 2: 354–86.

Skrabanek P., McCormack J. (1990). *Follies and Fallacies in Medicine*. Glasgow: Tarragon Press.

Stainton-Rogers W. (1991) *Explaining Health and Illness: An Exploration of Diversity*. Hertfordshire: Harvester Wheatsheaf.

Wallston K., Wallston B., DeVellis R. (1978). 'Development of the multi-dimensional health locus of control scales'. *Health Education Monographs* 6: 161–70.

Index

Abel, T. 66, 67
Acheson Report (1998) 7
activity: health beliefs in Ireland
    261–2, 264–6; LA21 action plan
    49–50
adolescent networks, sexual
    health promotion in Peru 157,
    161–79
age 6, 66, 161
ageing: health beliefs and alcohol
    240, 245, 246; perceptions about
    health behaviours in Ireland
    254–67
ageing populations 4
agency 3, 7–8; adolescent 169–73,
    177, 178; and structure 8–9, 11
Agenda 21 21–2, 38–51; links with
    health promotion 41–3; Local
    Agenda 21 44–51; UK response
    43–4
Ajzen, I. 4
alcohol health education 159,
    231–52
alcohol misuse 13
Alma Ata Declaration on Primary
    Health Care (1978) 1, 88
Altman, D. 146
Anderson, K. 55
architecture,
    modernist/postmodernist 86–7
Association for Public Health
    conference, 1997 49
audit, as research tool, 31, 32
Australia, HIV testing rates 118–19
autonomy 8

Bacon, Francis 85
Bandura, A. 4, 249
Barnett, E. 201
barrier model of health behaviour
    in heavy drinkers 243–51
baseline survey: formative
    evaluation of sexual health
    promotion for gay men 108–9,
    115; peer-led HIV prevention in
    London 217, 218, 223–8, 229
Bauman, Z. 89
Baxter, T. 146
Becker, M. 4, 150
Beeken, S. 201
Bem, D. 4
Berkman, L. 55
Berman, M. 87
Berne–Munich lifestyle panel 67–73
Bernstein, R. 87
biomedical model 44, 48; early
    lifestyle approaches 55; and
    implementation of policy in
    Norway 128, 132–9 passim;
    postmodernism as corrective to
    79, 83–98
biomedicine, health beliefs in
    Ireland 159–60, 254–5
Birmingham Untreated Heavy
    Drinkers Project 159, 231–52
Blaxter, M. 56–7, 256, 264
Bonell, C. 103
Bourdieu, Pierre 61–2, 64, 70
Brännström, I. 11
breast-feeding see infant feeding
    behaviour

Breslow, L. 55
Bromley, D. 258
Brown, M. 90
Brundtland Report 39
Bunton, R. 4
Burke, M. 90
Burrows, R. 6, 9, 97

Camden, LA21 44
Camden and Islington Community
    Health Services NHS Trust, Gay
    Men's HIV Prevention Team
    213, 214, 216
cancer prevention 151
Castelli, W. 55
Castongs, C. 129
Catania, J. 108
causality/intertextuality 92–3, 96
census, used in formative evaluation
    106–8
Centre for Reviews and
    Dissemination, York 9
Chapman, S. 11
Charlton, B. 9, 83, 91
'Children by Choice, not Chance'
    initiative 179n2
Christiansen, T. 57
Coates, R. 108
Coates, T. 106
Cochrane Collaboration (1993) 9,
    86, 95, 209
Cohen, D. 6, 143, 150
community: healthy, effect on
    economic and social
    development 34; participation in
    Agenda 21 21, 22, 40–1, 44,
    46–7, 51
community development 8
community health promotion 1, 2,
    51, 138, 265
community health promotion
    research 6, 11, 13; Norway
    130–1, 133–5, 136–9;
sexual health among gay men
    79–80, 102–21; young people's
    sexual health promotion in Peru
    157, 161–79

complementary medicine, Ireland
    254–5
Comte, Auguste 85
Conner, M. 199
constructivism 83, 98
consumer culture 4
consumption, Weber's concept of
    lifestyle 58–9, 61
control 8, 9; heavy drinking 242,
    246, 249; infant feeding decisions
    185, 186, 187, 189, 196–7, 198,
    200–1
controlled trial 209, 217, 229; see
    also randomised control trials
Corbin, J. 233
Cornwell, J. 264
correspondence analysis 68, 70–3,
    74
cost-effectiveness 5, 11, 32, 80–1
cost-effectiveness analysis 146–7,
    152
Craig, N. 6
Cretin, S. 149
Cribb, A. 147
critical theory 92
Crombie, H. 42
cultural determinants of health see
    socio-cultural determinants
cultural norms see socio-cultural
    norms
cyber technology 4

Dahlgren, G. 6
Dahrendorf, R. 59–60
Davison, L. 250
Dean, K. 4
debt payments from developing
    countries 42
decentralisation 125, 127
decision-making: community
    participation in Agenda 21 40;
    individual 81, 143, 150–2;
    research on levels of 31–2
    (Norway 80, 128–39)
deconstruction 92, 98
deductivism 85
Department of Health 14, 44, 48,
    231

Descartes, R. 85
development work, in evaluative
    research 104–6, 119
Devon County Council 49
diet, health beliefs in Ireland
    258–61, 264–6
disciplinarity/interdisciplinarity 94
disease 4; *see also* biomedical model
district health authorities 47–8
Dodds, J. 208, 224, 227, 228

Earth Summit, Rio 1992 21, 38
Eastern Europe 23, 24
Eco-Management and Audit
    Scheme (EMAS) 45
Economic and Social Research
    Institute (ESRI), Dublin 256
economic appraisal of health
    promotion 5–6, 80–1, 97,
    142–53; cost benefit analysis
    144–6, 153; cost effectiveness
    analysis 146–7, 152; cost
    minimisation analysis 148; cost
    utility analysis 147–8, 153;
    differential timing of costs and
    benefits 148–50
economic determinants of health
    see socio-economic determinants
economic development *see* socio-
    economic development
economic policy, effect on health
    41–3
education: work of LA21 46, 48; *see
    also* health education
effectiveness 5, 9–10, 11, 103, 106,
    119, 120, 152; postmodernist
    approach to debate on 79,
    83–98; *see also* evaluation;
    outcome evaluation
efficiency as criterion 142, 143
Elmore, R. 129
empowerment 2, 95, 138–9
English Health Education
    Authority 251
Enlightenment 84, 86, 87
environment, implications of
    Agenda 21 for health promotion
    21–2, 38–51

environmental determinants of
    health 1, 2, 6, 14, 41, 48, 265
environmental health problems,
    Norway 130–1, 133, 135–7, 138
Epi-Centre 9, 209, 229
Ershoff, D. 144
ethnicity, and infant feeding 185
evaluation 10, 11–15, 84, 209;
    economic *see* economic
    appraisal; Gay Men's Task Force
    initiative 79–80, 102–21; HIV
    prevention among gay men
    209–10, 216–29; language 97
Evang, Karl 126
Evans, R. 6
evidence: evaluation of Gay Men's
    Task Force initiative 102–21;
    meaning of 3, 9–15;
    postmodernist approach 83–98
experience, as source of health
    education 237–40, 246
experimental methods 9–15, 85–6,
    91, 95–6, 105–6; *see also*
    randomised control trials

Field, K. 146
Finland, infant feeding 184
Fishbein, M. 4
folk medicine, Ireland 160, 254–5
Folklore Commission of Ireland
    254
formative evaluation 79–80, 103,
    105, 106–12, 119, 120
Foucault, M. 5, 165
foundationalism 94
France: lay representation of health
    250–1; older people's
    representation of lifestyle 256,
    266; urban development 86
Fraser, E. 13
Freed, G. 201, 202

gay men: HIV prevention in
    London 158, 207–29; sexual
    health promotion in Scotland
    79–80, 102–21
Gay Men's HIV Prevention Team
    213, 214, 216

Gay Men's Sexual Health Survey 207–8, 224
Gay Men's Task Force initiative 79–80, 102–21
gender 6, 66
gendered space, and sexual health promotion in Peru 157, 161–79
Germany, health related lifestyles 67–73
Giddens, A. 4, 8, 9, 58
Gillies, P. 4, 7, 96
Gilson, G. 50
Giugliani, E. 201
Glanz, K. 232
global/local 38–51
globalisation 4, 23, 42, 87–8
'Going for Green' initiative 43
Good, C. 254
governance: and policy 3, 4–6; research into decision-making levels 31–2
Graham, H. 250, 265
Greece, infant feeding behaviour 158, 185, 187–203
Griffiths, W. 231
grounded theory analysis 159, 233
group, limits of earlier lifestyle approaches 55–6
Gulino, C. 187, 201

Habermas, J. 85, 87, 164, 165
habitus (Bourdieu) 61–2, 64–5
Hall, P. 44
Haraway, D. 90
Harry, J. 107
Hart, G. 107
Harvey, D. 87, 89, 90
Hawe, P. 6
Haycox, A. 147
Hayes, M. 90, 96
Hays, R. 106
health: as investment 21, 25–34; lay representation 250–1; as opposite of disease see biomedical model; postmodern view 88, 89; as resource for living 88, 157, 166, 167
health action zones 9

health behaviours: harm reduction behaviours of heavy drinkers 159, 243, 246; Ireland 159–60, 254–67; and lifestyle 55–75; see also individual behaviour change; psycho-social models; risk behaviour
Health Belief Model 185, 186, 249
health beliefs: heavy drinkers 240–1, 245, 246; infant feeding 158, 186–203 passim; Ireland 159–60, 254–67
health care: changes 1, 6; evaluating see economic appraisal; evaluation
health development 2
health-directed behaviour, distinguished from health-related behaviour 255, 266
health economics see economic appraisal
health education: for heavy drinkers 159, 231–52; infant feeding beliefs 158, 199–200
Health Education Authority 38, 96
Health for All 2000 Strategy 1, 26, 41, 45, 94, 127, 166
health impact assessments 50
health improvement 9, 13, 21; programmes 9, 48; see also Investment for Health approach
health indicators 13–14, 50–1, 74, 94–5, 96–7
health inequalities 3, 6–7, 8, 21, 24, 41, 44, 54, 56
health information: sexual, Peru 171–3, 174; see also health education
health intentions: heavy drinkers 250, 251; infant feeding 158, 185, 186, 187, 192, 198, 199, 200; and lifestyles 63
Health of the Nation white paper (DoH) 44, 47–8, 231
health oriented lifestyles 63–5, 67–73
health professionals: health

education by 237–8; and infant feeding 189, 194, 195, 196, 200–1

health promotion: attitudes of older people in Ireland 261, 265–6; benefits, evaluation of 145–6, 149–52; developments 1–2; endpoints of 6, 13; implications of postmodernism for 91–5; infrastructure 2, 31; links with sustainable development 41–3, 47–50

health promotion assets, research on 33

health promotion policy: Norway 80, 125–39; relationship to health promotion practice and research 1–15, 265, 266; research implications of recent changes 21, 23–34

health promotion practice 27, 157–60; postmodern approach 95–7; relationship to health promotion policy and research 1–15, 265, 266

health promotion research: definition 2–3; implications of Investment for Health approach for 21, 28–34; and LA21 50–1; lifestyle 22, 54–75; meaning of evidence 3, 9–15; nature of knowledge 3–9; postmodern approach 95–7; *see also* methodology

health promotion theory 1, 4, 8, 11, 15, 21–2; *see also* implementation theory; postmodernism; sociological theory

health-related behaviour, distinguished from health-directed behaviour 255, 266

health related lifestyles: distinguished from health oriented lifestyles 63; future research directions 73–5; new theoretical concept 63–6; patterns of behaviours and orientations in Berne–Munich

lifestyle panel 67–73; structure of 66–7; theoretical criteria 58–62

health services 1; and health promotion in Norway 80, 126–39; and infant feeding 189–90, 196–7, 200–1

Health 21 21, 26

healthism 266

healthy alliances 44, 47, 48, 94

Healthy Cities initiatives 45, 47, 94

healthy living centres 9, 231

heart, disease and health 5, 11, 93

Helsing, E. 201

hepatitis B 116, 118, 119

Herzlich, C. 251, 256

Hickson, F. 107, 208, 227

HIV infection: gay men 104, 108, 116–19, 120; risk reduction 158–9, 207–29

HIV testing 116, 118–19, 225, 226, 227, 228

Holsti, O. 258

Hope, V. 107

Howard, F. 201

Huberman, M. 131

Huyssens, A. 89

identity 8

illness, responses to, in Ireland 159–60, 254–5, 258–66

implementation theory 80, 128–39

Independent Inquiry into Inequalities in Health (Acheson Report) 7

individual behaviour change 44, 48, 231; gay men 107, 115–19, 208–29; *see also* lifestyle approach; lifestyles

individual health promotion 1, 2, 3; decision-making 81, 143, 150–2; *see also* individual behaviour change

inductivism 85

Ineichen, B. 185, 201

infant feeding behaviour 157–8, 183–203

information technology 4

International Health Promotion

Conference, 1st, Ottawa 1986 1,
    2, 5; *see also* Ottawa charter
International Health Promotion
    Conference, Adelaide 2
International Health Promotion
    Conference, Sundsvall 2
International Health Promotion
    Conference, 4th, Jakarta 1–2; *see
    also* Jakarta Declaration
international health promotion
    policy *see* World Health
    Organization
Internet 8
intersubjectivity 164–6
intervention utility 80, 120
interview study, health beliefs in
    Ireland 159–60, 254–67
Investment for Health approach 21,
    25–8; research implications
    28–34
Ireland, health beliefs, behaviours
    and response to illness 159–60,
    254–67

Jakarta Declaration (World Health
    Organization 1997) 1–2, 26, 88
Jameson, F. 89
Jan, S. 147
Japan, infant feeding 199
Jencks, C. 87
Jewish mothers 185

Kauth, M. 108
Kawachi, I. 51
Keeler, E. 149
Kegeles, S. 117
Kelleher, C. 255
Kelly, J. 106, 107, 116, 210, 211, 221
Kelly, M. 9
Kelly, P. 83, 91, 97
Kickbusch, I. 26, 66
Kippax, S. 116, 117
Kitson, A. 14
knowledge, nature of 3–9
Kohlmann, T. 66
Kooiker, S. 57
Korkia, P. 213
Krippendorf, K. 258

Labonte, R. 6, 41, 93
Labour Government 48
Lalonde Report (1974) 1, 88
Lancashire County Council 49–50
Lazarro, E. 201
Leibniz, G.W.von 85
life expectancy 7, 24, 42, 264
lifestyle approach 22, 54–75; earlier
    approaches 55–7; empirical
    findings 66–7; future directions
    in research 73–5; methodology
    66–73, 74; new concept of health
    related lifestyles 63–6;
    theoretical definitions 58–66
lifestyle effect 146
lifestyles 25, 48; and health in
    Ireland 159, 256–67; responses
    to health education messages
    from Birmingham Untreated
    Heavy Drinkers Cohort 231–52
Littman, H. 202
Liverpool, LA21 44
Local Agenda 21 (LA21) movement
    9, 22, 39, 44–50; health
    promotion research and 50–1
local authorities: and Agenda 21 22,
    39, 43, 44–51; implementation of
    health promotion policy in
    Norway 80, 125–39
Local Food Links 49
Local Government Management
    Board 40, 45
local health strategies 47, 231
London: 4 gym health promotion
    project for gay men 158–9,
    212–29; HIV testing rates 118;
    LA21 44;
    modernism/postmodernism in
    urban development 87; sexual
    risk behaviour among gay men
    207–8, 211–29
London School of Economics 166
Lupton, D. 5
Lyotard, J. 84, 87

MacArthur, C. 107
Macdonald, G. 95
MacFarlane, A. 255

Macintyre, S. 54
Maiman, L. 150
Manstead, A. 187, 188, 189, 201
Marks, J. 144
McCluskey, D. 256, 264
McQueen, D. 8–9, 66
McVey, D. 4
media, and health education 237
medical pluralism 254
methodological pluralism 10–11,
    15, 98; evaluation of peer-led
    community-level intervention to
    promote sexual health among
    gay men 79–80, 102–21
methodology: challenges 6, 79–81;
    community-based sexual health
    promotion in Peru 157, 170,
    173–6, 177; health education
    study of heavy drinkers 233–7;
    health lifestyle research 66–73,
    74; hierarchy of evidence 9–15,
    95–6; HIV prevention among
    gay men 209, 216–23;
    implementation study, Norway
    130–1; modernist/postmodernist
    approach 83–98; social cognition
    study of infant feeding 187–90,
    199; study of health beliefs and
    behaviours in Ireland 256–8
Meyrick, J. 96
Milburn, K. 170, 179
Miles, M. 131
Miller, D. 256
Ministry of Agriculture, Food and
    Fisheries 49
modernism: approach to health
    promotion research 83–98; and
    governance 4–6
MONICA Project 55
Mooney, G. 147, 150
Morse, J. 258
mortality 7, 13, 24, 55, 264
multi-media technology in SaRA
    initiative in Peru 157, 170,
    173–6, 177
Murphy, A. 254, 255
Murphy, E. 96

Nardone, A. 107, 208, 224, 227, 228
narratives 8
National Food Alliance 49
National Programme for Health
    Promotion, Norway 80, 125–39
Neuberger, H. 149
NGOs 166, 171
Noack, H. 4
Norman, P. 199
Norton, J. 208
Norway, implementation evaluation
    of national programme of health
    promotion 80, 125–39
Nutbeam, D. 12, 13, 209

Oakley, Ann 12, 13, 106
objectivity/subjectivity 93–4
O'Campo, P. 184, 187
O'Cathain, S. 254, 255
openness 13
Opportunities for Change
    consultation document 44
Ottawa Charter (WHO 1986) 1, 23,
    24, 41, 88, 127, 128, 138, 265
Our Common Future (Brundtland
    Report) 39
Our Healthier Nation consultation
    paper 14, 44, 48, 231, 232
outcome evaluation 11, 14, 98; gay
    men in Scotland 80, 103–4,
    105–6, 115–20, 121; health
    economics 145–6, 150, 153;
    Norway's health promotion
    policy 131; peer-led HIV
    prevention in London 220–1,
    222

Parsonage, M. 149
participant observation 107
partnership approach 2, 13, 14, 51
Paterson, E. 256, 264
Pawson, N. 92, 129
peer-led interventions for gay men
    79–80, 102–21, 158, 207–29
Peru, young people's sexual health
    promotion 157, 161–79
phenomenology 79, 103
Phillips, C. 147

Platt, S. 4
Plymouth and Torbay Health
    Authority 49
Poland, B. 83
policy analysis 50
Popay, J. 8
positive health 13–14; key
    postmodern health promotion
    concept 91–2, 95
positivist/post-positivist paradigm
    79, 83–98, 103
postmodernism 79, 83–98;
    approach to health promotion
    research and practice 95–7;
    implications for health
    promotion 91–5; limits 89–91
prevention 3, 5
process evaluation 80, 98, 103, 104,
    105, 112–15, 119, 120, 121;
    Norwegian health promotion
    policy 80, 128–39; peer-led HIV
    prevention in London 221, 223
professional identity 12
psycho-social determinants of
    health 6, 7; health beliefs in
    Ireland 262–3, 264; lifestyle 56
psycho-social models of health
    behaviour 4, 150, 160; heavy
    drinkers 249–51; infant feeding
    185–202; sexual health
    promotion in Peru 161–79
public health 1, 2, 14, 24, 29, 32;
    Ireland 264; sustainable
    development in UK 44, 47–8, 49,
    51
Public Health Alliance 49
public policy 1, 2, 3, 21, 50, 265
Puska, P. 55
Putnam, R. 7, 51

qualitative/quantitative methods
    9–15; postmodern approach 91,
    95–6; *see also* methodology;
    randomised control trials

Radley, A. 255, 266
randomised control trials 10, 11, 12,
    13, 105–6, 121, 145, 209;

    postmodern approach 83, 86, 91,
    95
Ratcliffe, J. 146
rationality/irrationality 92–3
regeneration partnerships 9
Reid, D. 39, 145
Restrepo, Helena 14
Rio Earth Summit (1992) 21, 38
risk 4–5, 12
risk behaviour: gay men in London
    158–9, 207–8, 220–9; gay men in
    Scotland 104–21; gay men in
    USA 106, 209, 210–11, 229;
    health education for heavy
    drinkers 231, 232, 239–52;
    lifestyle approach 55, 56, 73–4
risk harm reduction 13, 29; peer
    education intervention for gay
    men in London 158–9, 207–29
Robertson, A. 93
Rogers, A. 9
Rogers, E. 4, 210
Rootman, I. 9, 12
Rosen, M. 146
Rosenau, P. 93
Rosenstock, I. 249

safer sex for gay men 106, 116–18,
    158, 215
St Lawrence, J. 106
Saltzman, S. 108
SaRA initiative 166–78; difficulties
    177–8; gendered spaces in
    practice 168–73; multi-media
    technologies 173–6
Sayer, A. 92
Scandinavia: infant feeding 184,
    187; lifestyle approach 55
Scotland: evaluation of peer-led
    community-level intervention to
    promote sexual health of gay
    men 79–80, 102–21; infant
    feeding behaviour 158, 183–4,
    187–203; links between
    sustainable development and
    health 49
Scottish Office, Department of
    Health 5, 14, 199

Seage, G. 108
Seedhouse, D. 4
self-administered questionnaires
    (SAQ) 107, 108–9, 110–11, 113,
    218–19, 223–8
self-efficacy 249
self-help movements 8
self-identity 8
sex education 13
sexual health promotion: gay men
    79–80, 102–21, 158–9, 207–29;
    young people in Peru 157,
    161–79
SHARE evaluation 13
Sheill, A. 6
Shoemaker, F. 4
Simmel, Georg 58
Slovenia 31
smoking 13, 66, 144, 146, 152, 250
social capital 7, 50–1
social care, changes 1
social cognition approach, infant
    feeding behaviour 157–8,
    183–203
social determinants of health *see*
    socio-economic determinants
social diffusion 145–6, 210
social inclusion 13
social interventions 12
social movements 8
social norms *see* socio-cultural
    norms
social structure *see* structure
socio-cultural determinants of
    health 3, 6, 14, 41, 88–9; lifestyle
    approach 56–75
socio-cultural norms: infant feeding
    158, 185, 186, 187, 189, 194–6,
    197, 198, 199, 201; Ireland 160,
    254, 265
socio-economic change 4, 23–4; and
    policy implementation in
    Norway 134–5
socio-economic determinants of
    health 2, 6–7, 14, 88–9; health
    beliefs in Ireland 256, 258–66;
    infant feeding decisions 190–2,
    198–9; and international policy

21, 23–8, 29–30, 33–4; lifestyle
    56–75, 252, 256; sustainable
    development 41–3, 48
socio-economic development,
    contribution of health to 25,
    33–4
socio-economic status 6–7, 56–7,
    58–61, 66; survey of health
    behaviours in Ireland 257
socio-environmental model of
    health 97
sociological theory, and lifestyle 22,
    54–75
Soil Association 49
Somers, M. 8
Springett, J. 129
Stainton-Rogers, W. 254
state: health promotion policy in
    UK 2, 3; health promotion
    policy in Norway 80, 125–39;
    response to Agenda 21 in UK
    43–4, 49
steroid use, 4 gym health promotion
    project 158–9, 213, 215, 220
Stevenson, H. 90
Stimson, G. 213
Stoddart, G. 6
Strauss, A. 233
structuration theory 9
structure 3; and agency 8–9, 11; and
    health in Norway 134–5; lifestyle
    approach 55–75; *see also* socio-
    economic determinants
surveillance 5
sustainability audits 45, 50
Sustainability Indicators 45–6
sustainability, sustainable
    development 21–2, 38–51; links
    with health promotion 41–3,
    47–50
*Sustainable Development: the UK
    Strategy* 43–4
Sweeney, M. 187, 201
Switzerland: health related lifestyles
    67–73

theoretical domains (Dean) 4
Theory of Reasoned Action and

Planned Behaviour 185–6, 190, 198
Tilley, R. 92, 129
time-related perceptions of health behaviour 159–60, 254–67
Tolley, K. 6, 149
Too Much Drink THINK campaign 251
Towards a Healthier Scotland white paper 14
town planning: positivist/post-positivist development 86–7; and sustainable development 48
traditional medicine, Ireland 160, 254–5
transparency 13

Uitenbroek, D. 66
unemployment 24, 49, 134
Unicef 202
United Kingdom: health promotion policy 2, 3, 5, 7, 9, 10, 13, 14, 44, 47–8, 49, 51; infant feeding 183–203; local health strategy 44–51; older people's representation of lifestyle 266; response to Agenda 21 43–4; *see also* Scotland
United Kingdom Health Promotion Research Conference, 1st, Edinburgh 1998 3
United Kingdom Health Promotion Research Conference, 2000 15
United Nations General Assembly 39
United States of America: infant feeding 199; lifestyle approaches in health research 55; sexual risk reduction among gay men 106, 209, 210–11, 229; urban development 86–7
universality and generalisability in research 94–5, 96–7
urban development, modernist/postmodernist 86–7

Utility Model of Preventive Behaviour 143, 151–2

Walker, D. 6
Wallston, K. 4
Walt, G. 50
Waterston, T. 201
Webb, D. 93, 97
Weber, Max 22, 58–61, 62, 63, 67–8
Weinstein, N. 249
well-being 95
West, R. 149
Whitehead, M. 6, 33
Whitelaw, A. 3, 4, 13
Wilkinson, R. 7, 33, 42, 51
Wilks, S. 44
Williams, A. 149
Williams, J. 4
Willms, S. 90, 96
Wimbush 103
Windsor, R. 144
World Bank 42
World Commission on Environment and Development 39
World Conservation Strategy 39
World Health Organization 1, 23, 88, 132, 138, 139; guidance on evaluation 12; Healthy Cities initiative 45, 47, 94; and infant feeding 183, 188, 202; MONICA Project 55; Regional Office for Europe's health promotion programme 21, 23–34, 41; *see also* Health for All 2000 Strategy; Jakarta Declaration; Ottawa Charter

Yeo, S. 199
Young, I. 90
Young, S. 48
young people, sexual health promotion in Peru 157, 161–79

Ziglio, E. 4